100 Questions & Answers About Liver, Heart, and Kidney Transplantation
A Lahey Clinic Guide

Hannah M. Gilligan, MD
Medical Director of Kidney Transplantation
Lahey Clinic Medical Center
Burlington, MA

David M. Venesy, MD
Director, Heart Failure Program
Director, Cardiac Care Unit
Lahey Clinic Medical Center, Burlington, MA
Staff Physician, Heart Failure and Cardiac Transplant Center
Tufts Medical Center
Assistant Professor of Medicine
Tufts University School of Medicine
Boston, MA

Fredric D. Gordon, MD
Medical Director of Liver Transplantation
Director of Hepatology
Lahey Clinic Medical Center, Burlington, MA
Assistant Professor of Medicine
Tufts Medical School
Boston, MA

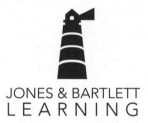

JONES & BARTLETT
L E A R N I N G

World Headquarters

Jones & Bartlett Learning	Jones & Bartlett Learning	Jones & Bartlett Learning
40 Tall Pine Drive	Canada	International
Sudbury, MA 01776	6339 Ormindale Way	Barb House, Barb Mews
978-443-5000	Mississauga, Ontario L5V 1J2	London W6 7PA
info@jblearning.com	Canada	United Kingdom
www.jblearning.com		

Jones & Bartlett Learning books and products are available through most bookstores and online booksellers. To contact Jones & Bartlett Learning directly, call 800-832-0034, fax 978-443-8000, or visit our website, www.jblearning.com.

Substantial discounts on bulk quantities of Jones & Bartlett Learning publications are available to corporations, professional associations, and other qualified organizations. For details and specific discount information, contact the special sales department at Jones & Bartlett Learning via the above contact information or send an email to specialsales@jblearning.com.

The authors, editor, and publisher have made every effort to provide accurate information. However, they are not responsible for errors, omissions, or for any outcomes related to the use of the contents of this book and take no responsibility for the use of the products and procedures described. Treatments and side effects described in this book may not be applicable to all people; likewise, some people may require a dose or experience a side effect that is not described herein. Drugs and medical devices are discussed that may have limited availability controlled by the Food and Drug Administration (FDA) for use only in a research study or clinical trial. Research, clinical practice, and government regulations often change the accepted standard in this field. When consideration is being given to use of any drug in the clinical setting, the health care provider or reader is responsible for determining FDA status of the drug, reading the package insert, and reviewing prescribing information for the most up-to-date recommendations on dose, precautions, and contraindications, and determining the appropriate usage for the product. This is especially important in the case of drugs that are new or seldom used.

Production Credits
Executive Publisher: Christopher Davis
Editorial Assistant: Sara Cameron
Associate Production Editor: Leah Corrigan
Associate Marketing Manager: Katie Hennessy
Manufacturing and Inventory Supervisor: Amy Bacus
Composition: Glyph International
Cover Designer: Carolyn Downer
Cover images: (top) © Kimberly Anne Reinick/ShutterStock, Inc., (bottom left)
© Yuri Arcurs/ShutterStock, Inc., (bottom right) © SpastMedia/ShutterStock, Inc.
Printing and Binding: Malloy, Inc.
Cover Printing: Malloy, Inc.

Library of Congress Cataloging-in-Publication Data
Gilligan, Hannah M.
  100 questions and answers about liver, heart, and kidney transplantation : a Lahey Clinic guide /
Hannah M. Gilligan, David M. Venesy, Fredric D. Gordon.
    p. cm.
  Includes index.
  ISBN 978-0-7637-8609-0 (alk. paper)
  1. Kidneys—Transplantation—Miscellanea. 2. Kidneys—Transplantation—Popular works.
3. Liver—Transplantation—Miscellanea. 4. Liver—Transplantation—Popular works.
5. Heart—Transplantation—Miscellanea. 6. Heart—Transplantation—Popular works.
I. Venesy, David M. II. Gordon, Fredric D. III. Title. IV. Title: One hundred questions and
answers about liver, heart, and kidney transplantation.
  RD575.G55 2011
  617.4'610592—dc22
                                    2010018001

6048

Printed in the United States of America
14 13 12 11 10   10 9 8 7 6 5 4 3 2 1

This book is dedicated to my father, Thomas J. Gilligan, Jr., MD, who was my first teacher.

—Hannah M. Gilligan, MD

This book is dedicated both to my mom, Barbara Venesy, whose unwavering pursuit of excellence has inspired all of us to be our very best, and to my beautiful wife, Lora, whose incredible love and support, as well as her encouragement of my academic and clinical pursuits, has been my rock. Lora's ardent passion for life and boundless compassion has inspired me to be a better doctor, and to be a better person.

—David M. Venesy, MD

This book is dedicated to my parents, Harriet and Alan Gordon, who taught me the value of education, perseverance, and compassion.

—Fredric D. Gordon, MD

Contents

Ever since the first kidney transplant was performed in 1954, transplantation has become an essential, life-saving procedure for people with organ failure. Currently there are over 100,000 people in the United States waiting for organ transplantation. The vast majority, over 83,000, is awaiting kidney transplantation; almost 16,000 are awaiting liver transplantation and over 3,000 are awaiting heart transplantation. Fortunately, organ transplantation remains an important issue in the nation's social and political consciousness.

The success of organ transplantation has also grown steadily since its inception. These improvements are attributable to advances in surgical technique, pharmaceuticals, and preoperative and postoperative care. Organ recipients can now expect longer and healthier lives.

This book is written for patients awaiting kidney, liver, or heart transplantation and their families to help navigate through the transplant system. *100 Questions & Answers About Liver, Heart, and Kidney Transplantation: A Lahey Clinic Guide* demystifies the process so that patients can actively participate in their health care. It gives a brief overview of chronic kidney, liver, and heart diseases that necessitate transplantation. It is our hope that this book will be useful to transplant candidates as they initiate their evaluations, understand the complexity of organ allocation, address their complications during the waiting period, and ultimately undergo transplantation.

100 Questions & Answers About Liver, Heart, and Kidney Transplantation: A Lahey Clinic Guide also addresses the field of living donor adult transplantation for kidney and liver candidates. Given the national shortage of donated organs, living donor transplantation may be the only real option for a growing proportion of the candidates on the waiting list. The number of organ donors grew steadily through the 1990s but seems to have plateaued at approximately

28,000 annually for the past five years. New ways to expand the donor pool are addressed in our book.

For the patient who has been fortunate enough to receive a transplant, this book will be helpful. It reviews the immunosuppressive medications (indications and potential adverse effects). It describes long-term expectations, for example, graft survival rates. We discuss potential complications and ways to preserve your transplant function.

We hope that our book will help answer your questions and make you an active participant in the transplant process.

Hannah M. Gilligan, MD
David M. Venesy, MD
Fredric D. Gordon, MD

Renal Transplantation

PART ONE

The Basics

What is renal failure?

What causes chronic kidney disease?

How long can I live on dialysis?

More . . .

1. What is renal failure?

Kidneys

Two bean-shaped organs located on either side of your spine that regulate the excretion of waste products and fluids, balance chemicals and minerals, and secrete hormones that affect the body's ability to produce red blood cells and affect your blood pressure.

The **kidneys** are two bean-shaped organs located on either side of your spine under your lowest ribs. The kidneys have three major roles:

1. They regulate the excretion of waste products and fluids from the body.
2. They balance the chemicals and minerals in your body.
3. They secrete hormones that affect the body's ability to produce red blood cells (erythropoietin) and affect your blood pressure (renin).

Renal failure

When the kidneys can no longer provide their vital functions.

Renal failure occurs when the kidneys can no longer provide these vital functions. We begin to retain fluid and develop swollen legs. Our electrolytes are no longer in balance; for example, the potassium may be high. We become anemic because we no longer produce enough erythropoietin. We develop higher blood pressure. With advanced renal failure we fail to excrete toxins such as urea, which makes us feel ill (nausea, fatigue).

Creatinine

Blood test used as a marker of kidney function.

The **creatinine** is a blood test that we use as a marker of kidney function. It is a natural breakdown product of muscle that passes freely through the kidney; it is neither reabsorbed nor metabolized by the kidney so it gives us information about the function of the kidneys. A normal creatinine is less than or equal to 1.3 mg/dL for men and less than 1.1 mg/dL for women.

2. Can you tell me what CKD means?

CKD is chronic kidney disease. We classify the degree of chronic kidney disease into stages or degrees of severity (**Table 1**).

Glomerular filtration rate

Measure of the kidney's ability to filter. It gives us an estimate of what kind of a job your kidneys are doing.

GFR is **glomerular filtration rate**. This is a measure of the kidney's ability to filter. It gives us an estimate

Table 1   Stage of Chronic Kidney Disease

Stage 1	GFR > 90 mL/min	Kidney damage with normal or high GFR.
Stage 2	GFR 60 to 89 mL/min	Kidney damage with mild decrease in GFR.
Stage 3	GFR 30 to 59 mL/min	Moderate decrease in GFR.
Stage 4	GFR 15 to 29 mL/min	Severe decrease in GFR.
Stage 5	GFR < 15 mL/min	Kidney failure (ESRD).

Source: KDOQI CKD Classification.

of what kind of a job your kidneys are doing. There are various methods for measuring the GFR. Your nephrologist may ask you to collect your urine for 24 hours. The urine and serum creatinine concentrations are measured. Using a mathematical formula with urine creatinine and serum creatinine, we can determine your GFR. There are more scientific methods (inulin clearance, iothalamate clearance) to measure kidney filtration, but they are not widely used in clinical practice.

ESRD is **end-stage renal disease**. End-stage renal disease signals that the kidneys can no longer provide their vital functions, which include excreting toxins, managing electrolytes, and maintaining a proper fluid balance. The GFR is less than 15 mL/min when ESRD occurs.

End-stage renal disease

Signals that the kidneys can no longer provide their vital functions, which include excreting toxins, managing electrolytes, and maintaining a proper fluid balance.

3. What causes chronic kidney disease?

The most common cause of chronic kidney disease in the United States is diabetic kidney disease, called diabetic nephropathy. The second most common cause of chronic kidney disease in the United States is hypertension-related renal disease, referred to as hypertensive nephrosclerosis. These are secondary causes of chronic kidney disease where a particular disease is damaging the kidneys. Diabetes and hypertension are the most well-known causes of chronic kidney disease, but there are many others.

Primary causes of chronic kidney disease are diseases that solely affect the kidneys. For example, chronic glomerulonephritis such as IgA nephropathy is the most common form of primary chronic kidney disease in the world. Chronic glomerulonephritis causes inflammation that attacks the kidneys. There are numerous examples of primary causes of chronic kidney disease.

4. My nephrologist (kidney specialist) sent me a letter that my serum creatinine is 3.0 mg/dL and I have stage 3 CKD. What does this mean?

Stage 3 CKD indicates a moderate decrease in GFR. At this stage of CKD, we start to see problems related to the decline in renal function. Your nephrologist will start to look for potential renal-related issues such as higher blood pressure, anemia (low red blood cell count), electrolyte abnormalities (high potassium, high phosphorus), and fluid retention (weight gain or swelling in the legs). It's time to start thinking about renal replacement therapy.

Transplantation

Surgical procedure in which a healthy organ from another person (donor) is placed into your body to assume the work of your non-functioning organ.

Dialysis

A life-sustaining treatment that literally takes over the job of your kidneys. The two major types of dialysis are hemodialysis and peritoneal dialysis.

Renal replacement therapy is just as it sounds: It is therapy that is going to replace or take over the job of your kidneys. There are two types of renal replacement therapy: transplantation and dialysis.

Transplantation is a surgical procedure in which a healthy kidney from another person (donor) is placed into your body to assume the work of your nonfunctioning kidneys. **Dialysis** is a life-sustaining treatment. Dialysis literally takes over the job of your kidneys. There are two major types of dialysis: hemodialysis and peritoneal dialysis.

Hemodialysis involves a dialysis machine with a filter that "cleans" your blood by removing toxins, correcting your electrolytes and removing excess fluid from your body. Typically, you attend an outpatient dialysis center three times a week for your dialysis treatment. Most treatments last between 3 and 4 hours.

During a dialysis treatment blood is removed from your body and pumped through a dialysis filter. The "cleaned" blood is returned to your body. To perform dialysis we need access to your blood supply. A catheter (a tube) can be placed in a large vein in your body, such as the jugular vein in your neck, subclavian vein in your chest, or femoral vein in your groin. The catheter has two ports, one for removing blood to go through the dialysis filter and one to return the "clean" blood to your body. A catheter is a temporary access.

A permanent access is an arteriovenous fistula. A surgeon performs an operation to attach a vein and an artery in your arm to form an arteriovenous fistula. If your veins are small, an alternative access is a graft. A surgeon performs an operation using a soft tube to link an artery and vein together. The fistula and graft are both under the skin. They look like large veins. The dialysis staff is able to access the fistula or graft by placing two needles. The needles are connected to tubing. One needle draws blood from the fistula or graft and the blood is pumped through the dialysis filter. The "clean" blood is then returned via the second needle to the patient.

In **peritoneal dialysis** your peritoneal membrane (the covering of your abdominal organs) acts as a filter. A catheter is placed into your abdominal cavity. You fill the abdominal cavity with peritoneal dialysis fluid.

The Basics

Hemodialysis
A process in which a dialysis machine with a filter "cleans" your blood by removing toxins, correcting your electrolytes and removing excess fluid from your body.

Peritoneal dialysis
A process by which your peritoneal membrane (the covering of your abdominal organs) acts as a filter. The abdominal cavity is filled with peritoneal dialysis fluid. The peritoneal membrane filters toxins and fluids from your blood into the peritoneal dialysis fluid. The peritoneal fluid containing the toxins is drained from your body after several hours and replaced with fresh peritoneal dialysis fluid. This procedure is called an exchange.

The peritoneal membrane filters toxins and fluids from your blood into the peritoneal dialysis fluid. The peritoneal fluid containing the toxins is drained from your body after several hours and replaced with fresh peritoneal dialysis fluid. This procedure is called an exchange.

In continuous ambulatory peritoneal dialysis, you will perform on average four exchanges in a 24-hour period, 7 days a week. In automated peritoneal dialysis, a cycler machine performs the exchanges automatically while you are sleeping.

5. I had a fistula placed 3 months ago. My vascular surgeon says it is mature and ready to be used. How will I know when I need to start hemodialysis?

You will be closely monitored by your nephrologist. Your nephrologist looks for any symptoms of renal failure, such as nausea or vomiting, increased sleepiness, difficulty concentrating, or twitching. Your nephrologist will assess your fluid status. Are you retaining fluid in your legs or lungs? Are you short of breath or having chest pain? Your nephrologist will review your blood work to be sure your kidneys are adequately maintaining your electrolytes and filtering toxins from your blood. Most patients need to start renal replacement therapy when they reach CKD stage 5. Some patients need to start renal replacement therapy at earlier stages depending on their symptoms, fluid status, and blood work.

6. How long can I live on dialysis?

It depends on many factors. In theory you can live many years on dialysis. There are patients who live over 30 years on dialysis; unfortunately, they are the exception.

Many of the diseases that predispose you to end-stage renal disease are associated with shortened life spans. It is not typically the dialysis that attenuates your life span but the reason you ended up on dialysis. Over many years dialysis access can become problematic. Accesses may become infected or stop working. This also can affect your longevity. The 5-year mortality rate for dialysis patients is 50%.

7. What happens if I decide against renal replacement therapy?

When you reach the point where you need renal replacement therapy (your kidneys are no longer able to provide their vital functions), if you choose not to have renal replacement therapy, you will die from uremia. Many factors determine your life span, for example, if you still make urine or if your potassium level runs high. However, most patients die within 2 weeks.

The Basics

PART TWO

Before
Transplantation

Why should I get a kidney transplant?
Am I even eligible?

What is involved in an evaluation
for kidney transplantation?

What can I do to expedite my evaluation
and move forward with my transplant?

More . . .

8. Why should I get a kidney transplant? Am I even eligible?

Patients with kidney transplants live longer than patients on dialysis. Most kidney transplant recipients report a better quality of life than on dialysis. It gives you an opportunity to live a more normal life.

Talk with your nephrologist about referring you to a kidney transplant program for evaluation. Patients on dialysis or patients with advanced chronic kidney disease (creatinine clearance less than 30 mL/min) can be evaluated for transplantation.

9. Are there any contraindications to kidney transplantation?

There are some absolute and relative contraindications to kidney transplantation. Absolute contraindications include

- Insufficient cardiac reserve
- Active cancer; untreated or progressive
- Ongoing illicit substance abuse
- Uncontrolled serious psychiatric illness
- Active infection
- Anatomy that does not make transplant technically possible

Relative contraindications include

- History of noncompliance with medical management; patient must demonstrate compliance for a specified period of time before consideration for transplantation
- History of cancer with no active disease at this time; decided on a case-by-case basis
- History of infection; must be free of infection at the time of transplantation

- Pregnancy
- Morbid obesity; body mass index greater than 40
- History of substance abuse
- Age equal to or over 80 years of age

Please speak directly with your proposed transplant center before you decide that you are not a candidate. Everyone who is interested in receiving a renal transplant should undergo an evaluation. Renal transplant programs can vary in what they consider a relative contraindication.

10. What is involved in an evaluation for kidney transplantation?

The evaluation begins when your nephrologist refers you to a kidney transplant program for an evaluation. The evaluation is necessary to learn about the risks and benefits of transplantation for each patient. It is an opportunity to review your medical history and identify any potential problems that need further investigation. It is also an opportunity for you to learn about renal transplantation.

The evaluation involves meeting the members of the transplant team who will assess you. The transplant nephrologist (a medical physician with expertise in kidney disease and caring for kidney patients before and after transplantation) reviews the evaluation process with you, including the risks and benefits of transplantation. The transplant nephrologist reviews your medical history, examines you, and answers any questions.

The other members of the team include a dietitian, who reviews your nutrition history and plans a diet to help you prepare for transplantation. The social worker interviews you to determine if you have any special concerns about the process and have adequate support after your transplant. An infectious disease physician reviews your history of infections and your immunization history. The infectious disease physician determines if you are free of active infection and if we can anticipate any particular infections after transplant. Our financial coordinator discusses any insurance concerns you may have and any financial programs available to you. Our transplant surgeon explains in detail the risks and benefits of the surgery. The surgeon assesses whether it is technically possible to perform the surgery.

Throughout the process, our transplant nurse coordinator supports you and expedites your evaluation. The transplant nurse coordinator is an invaluable resource. She or he is your main contact at the transplant center. The transplant nurse coordinator also starts your formal education about kidney transplantation.

After meeting the members of the team, you will have some blood labs drawn and some diagnostic studies ordered. The screening laboratory tests include

- Complete blood count
- INR and partial prothrombin time
- Basic metabolic profile
- Liver function studies
- Glycosylated hemoglobin (patients with diabetes or suspected)
- Urinalysis with culture and sensitivity (if patient makes urine)
- ABO blood group (measured on two separate occasions)
- CMV, EBV, HSV, and varicella titers (viral studies)
- HIV (AIDS test)
- Hepatitis studies

- Quantiferon gold test (for tuberculosis)
- Twenty-four–hour urine for protein and creatinine clearance (or calculated GFR) for patients not on dialysis

Other diagnostic studies include (as required)

- Chest x-ray
- ECG (electrocardiogram)
- Renal ultrasound of native kidneys
- Cardiac evaluation for patients over 50 years of age (preferably a dobutamine stress test)
- High-risk patients (positive stress test, history of coronary artery disease, congestive heart failure, long history of diabetes mellitus, sedentary lifestyle) referred for cardiac consultation
- Dental letter (to demonstrate no active disease)
- Cancer screening as recommended by the American Cancer Society to include updated prostate-specific antigen (PSA), Pap, mammogram, and colonoscopy

Other diagnostic studies that may be needed depending on the patient's history include

- Pulmonary function studies
- Carotid Doppler
- Cardiac catheterization
- Voiding cystourethrogram (this is a test to study your bladder and how well it is working)
- Lower extremity arterial vascular studies

After your evaluation is complete your information is presented to the multidisciplinary transplant team selection committee. The purpose of the screening meetings is to review data accumulated during your outpatient evaluation process to determine the appropriateness of transplantation for each patient. Final decisions reached by the committee include accept and activate for transplantation, accept but not activate, or decision deferred or the patient is not considered an appropriate candidate for kidney transplantation. The patient is notified of his or her status within 10 business days from the selection committee's meeting.

11. What can I do to expedite my evaluation and move forward with my transplant?

Have your medical records sent ahead to the transplant center. Bring in an updated medication list. Every transplant candidate is expected to be up to date with their preventive care. This would include vaccinations, colonoscopy (if you are over 50 years old), prostate-specific antigen (PSA) for men (over 50 years old), Pap smears for women, and mammograms for women over 40 years old. Start making appointments or talk with your primary care physician about getting your preventive care up to date. Bring someone with you to the evaluation. Bring your questions with you.

PART THREE

Organ Allocation

I heard there is a waiting list for kidney transplants. How do I get my name on the list?

How are a deceased donor and recipient matched?

How long will I need to wait for a transplant?

More . . .

12. I heard there is a waiting list for kidney transplants. How do I get my name on the list?

There is a waiting list for deceased donor transplants. A deceased donor kidney transplant is a kidney that comes from a brain-dead donor or a cadaver. Patients are listed according to their blood group: A, O, B, or AB. When the patient at the top of the list gets a kidney transplant, everyone moves up the list.

When you have completed your transplant evaluation and been accepted as a kidney transplant candidate, your transplant program activates you on the national waiting list.

Your HLAs are identified and entered onto a regional and national list. **HLA** stands for human leukocyte antigens, and these antigens are on leukocytes (white blood cells) and most solid tissues and organs of the body but are not present on red blood cells. They have many functions, but with regard to kidney transplantation they are the structures on the donor's kidney that the recipients recognize as different from themselves and try to destroy. If donor and recipient have the same HLAs, there is less chance that recipients will reject the kidney. Children of the same parents have a one chance in four of having exactly the same HLAs.

If a deceased donor kidney becomes available, the potential recipient is "crossmatched" with that donor. **Crossmatch** means that serum from the recipient (the clear liquid portion of the blood) is mixed with leukocytes from the donor in a test tube and allowed to react. The cells, which have the same antigens as the kidney to be transplanted, are then checked to be sure they have not been harmed by anything in the recipient's serum. If the cells are not harmed, the crossmatch

HLA

These antigens are on leukocytes (white blood cells) and most solid tissues and organs of the body but are not present on red blood cells. They are the structures on the donor's transplanted organ that the recipients recognize as different from themselves and try to destroy. If donor and recipient have the same HLAs, there is less chance of rejection.

Crossmatch

A test that determines whether recipient cells and donor cells are compatible, carried out before transplant can take place.

is said to be "compatible" and the kidney can be transplanted. If the cells have been harmed, the crossmatch is said to be "incompatible" and, in most cases, the transplant cannot happen.

Your blood type, tissue type, blood antibody levels, and body size are data entered into the waiting list computer program.

13. How are a deceased donor and recipient matched?

The following factors are taken into account when forming a match between donor and recipient:

- Blood type
- Tissue type
- Height and weight of transplant candidate
- Size of donated organ
- Time on the waiting list
- The distance between the donor and recipient hospitals
- The recipient transplant hospital's criteria for accepting organs

These factors are taken into account to get the most longevity out of an organ. Kidneys that share similar tissue typing characteristics tend to function for a longer period of time. Kidneys that are used locally limit the amount of time that the kidney remains outside the body. This also has been associated with better long-term outcomes.

After the match run (data about recipient and donor are entered into the computer), a donor and potential recipient are identified. Before moving ahead a crossmatch is done between the donor and recipient. If the crossmatch is negative (there was no reaction between the donor and recipient's cells), then the crossmatch can proceed. If the crossmatch is positive (if the cells between the donor and recipient are not compatible), then the transplant cannot take place because of the high probability that the recipient would reject (attack) the donor's kidney.

14. How long will I need to wait for a transplant?

That depends. The number of people waiting for a kidney transplant in October 2009 was 82,162. The number of kidney transplants from deceased donors performed this past year was 7,923 from January 1, 2009, through September 30, 2009.

Because of this large discrepancy between recipients and donors, ways to expand the donor pool are always sought. One way to expand the donor pool is to use living donors. From January 1, 2009, through September 30, 2009, there were 4,724 living donor kidney transplants performed in the United States. (More about living donors later.)

For many years only standard criteria donor kidneys were used for transplantation. A standard criteria donor kidney comes from a previously healthy individual between the age of 18 and 60 years of age who had an untimely death such as a motor vehicle accident. They were unable to survive their injuries and progressed to brain death. Their family made the generous offer to donate their organs.

Donation after cardiac death occurs when organs are donated from a patient on a ventilator who has severe brain injuries with no hope of meaningful recovery. Because of the futility of the patient's prognosis, the family makes the decision to withdraw ventilatory support. If the family elects to donate the patient's organs, the patient is taken to an operating room where the breathing tube is removed. If the patient's heart stops beating within 20 minutes, the transplant team can remove the kidneys. Kidneys from donation after cardiac death donors have similar outcomes (last as long and work as well) as standard criteria donor kidneys.

Research has shown that many less commonly used donor kidneys (such as a kidney from a donor older than 60 years of age) can benefit carefully selected candidates. The goal is to expand the donor pool and thereby shorten the wait time for kidney transplantation. This group of donors is called expanded criteria donors.

Selected candidates include but are not limited to patients who are having difficulty with their dialysis treatments and patients who may face a shorter life expectancy while on dialysis.

Candidates must give their written consent before being listed for an expanded criteria kidney transplantation. The consent form is reviewed with the transplant nephrologist or transplant surgeon. Candidates who agree to receive expanded criteria donor kidneys are also eligible to receive standard criteria donor kidneys.

Expanded criteria donors are over 60 years of age or between 50 and 59 years of age with one of these criteria:

- CVA (stroke) + HTN (hypertension) + Creat (creatinine) > 1.5 at the time of kidney placement
- CVA + HTN
- CVA + Creat > 1.5 at the time of kidney placement
- HTN + Creat > 1.5 at the time of kidney placement

- CVA = CVA was cause of death
- HTN = history of hypertension at any time

15. I have been unable to find a kidney donor. My nephrologist wants me to start dialysis, but I don't want to. Why can't I just put my name on the list and wait for a transplant to become available?

Unfortunately, the waiting time for a deceased donor kidney transplant can be years. Also, you do not receive waiting time unless you are on dialysis. You may be listed for a kidney transplant when your GFR is less than 20 mL/min but you will not receive any waiting time (so you will not advance up the waiting list). However, if a 6 antigen matched ("perfect") kidney became available, you would receive that kidney before everyone above you on the list. This is a rare occurrence, so you probably need to start dialysis while waiting for a kidney to become available.

PART FOUR

Living Donor Kidney Transplantation

Are there any other options for incompatible donors and recipients?

What makes a good donor? What if my living donor doesn't have health insurance?

My sister and I are being transplanted in 2 weeks. Our transplant nurse coordinator called today to arrange for our final crossmatch next week. Why do we have to repeat the crossmatch? We did it 3 months ago.

More . . .

16. I would rather have a transplant than go on dialysis. Is that possible? My brother has offered to be my donor. How do we get started?

You would start by having your nephrologist refer you to a kidney transplant program. At your first visit you are given information for any potential donors to call the live donor nurse coordinator. The live donor nurse coordinator briefly interviews your brother over the phone to make sure there were no obvious contraindications to donation and verify your donor's blood type.

When a person wishes to donate a kidney to a friend or relative, tests must be performed to be sure they are compatible. The first compatibility testing that is done is routine blood typing. This determines one set of antigens (chemical structures or molecules) that are present on red blood cells and also on all the body's tissues and organs, including the kidney. If a donor and recipient do not have compatible blood types, a very strong immune reaction (rejection) occurs, causing severe damage and generally loss of the kidney. Possible blood types are A, B, AB, or O. Recipients who are blood type O can only receive kidneys that are also blood type O. Recipients who are blood type AB may receive kidneys from all blood types. Recipients who are blood type A may receive kidneys from blood types A or O. Recipients who are blood type B may receive kidneys from blood types B or O. Blood type O is sometimes called the "universal donor" because it can be donated to all other blood types, whereas blood type AB is sometimes called the "universal recipient" because it can receive all other blood types.

As with deceased donor transplants, HLA testing is the second type of compatibility testing that is performed.

The crossmatch gives us a glimpse into the future of how your immune system would react to your brother's kidney.

You need to complete your transplant evaluation and be accepted to the deceased donor kidney transplant list before proceeding with live donation.

17. I heard some people talking at dialysis about doing a "swap." Can you explain that to me?

Because there is such a shortage of organs donated, there have been some innovative programs developed that use incompatible live donors and recipients. The "swap" that you are referring to is called a paired exchange. There are willing donors but they are unable to donate because their blood types are incompatible or their immune systems were incompatible (they had a positive crossmatch). In a **paired exchange** a donor and recipient are evaluated and accepted into a participating transplant program. Their information is entered into a computer. Match runs (a computer program that looks for compatible matches in the system) occur every 4 to 6 weeks. If there are any potential compatible pairs, the transplant programs are notified. They review the preliminary data of age, body mass index, and blood type and decide if they want to proceed. Crossmatch testing is done between the pairs, donors, and recipients. If the crossmatch is negative, the donors are further evaluated at the recipient's transplant hospital. A final crossmatch is done the week before surgery. If this continues to be negative, you proceed to transplantation. The surgery on the donors is performed simultaneously at the various transplant hospitals.

Paired exchange

A donor and recipient who are unable to donate because their blood types are incompatible or their immune systems were incompatible (they had a positive crossmatch) are evaluated and accepted into a participating transplant program to search for compatible matches.

18. My cousin and I have been in the paired exchange program for the last 4 months and have not had any matches. Is there another program available for incompatible living donors and recipients?

Another program for incompatible live donor and recipient is a list exchange. An incompatible living donor provides a kidney to the transplant hospital's deceased donor waiting list. In exchange, the recipient moves to the top of the region's waiting list for their ABO blood group. To be eligible for the list exchange, it must be the recipient's first deceased donor transplant. The recipient must be on dialysis and unsensitized (not have a high level of antibodies in their blood so that it would be difficult to match a kidney). The living donor and recipient must be on the paired exchange list for 90 days before moving to a list exchange.

Please check with your transplant program about paired and list exchanges because their exact qualifications may vary.

19. Are there any other options for incompatible donors and recipients?

Desensitization

A special medical treatment to try to remove donor-specific antibodies from the donor's blood whereby the recipient is treated with medication (intravenous immune globulin) to try to reduce the donor-specific antibodies.

Incompatible donors who have a positive crossmatch (antibodies in the recipient's blood that are directed against antigens on the donor's cells) can undergo special medical treatment to try to remove the donor-specific antibodies from the donor's blood. This process is called **desensitization**. The recipient is first treated with medication (intravenous immune globulin) to try to reduce the donor-specific antibodies. After this treatment the crossmatch is repeated. If it becomes negative, the transplant is performed within 3 to 5 days. If it is still positive, the donor can undergo a procedure called plasmapheresis. This is a treatment similar to hemodialysis in that the recipient's blood is pumped through a filter. In plasmapheresis the filter removes antibodies. After three plasmapheresis treatments the crossmatch is repeated. If it becomes negative, the transplant is performed within 3 to 5 days. If it remains positive, the medication and the plasmapheresis series may be repeated.

Desensitization is reserved for very specific circumstances. Patients who have high levels of antibodies in their blood and have been unable to find a compatible donor may be candidates for desensitization.

20. What makes a good donor? What if my living donor doesn't have health insurance?

A good donor is someone who comes forward freely to donate his or her kidney. They must be in excellent health with two normally functioning kidneys. They are carefully evaluated by members of the transplant team (the nephrologist and surgeon have not evaluated the recipient). We want to try to uncover any potential problems that the donor may have in the foreseeable future that would jeopardize their remaining kidney. Two such examples are diabetes mellitus and hypertension, which are the primary and secondary causes of end-stage renal disease in the United States.

Your insurance covers the cost of the donor's care related to transplant. The sale of organs is illegal in the United States.

21. My sister and I are being transplanted in 2 weeks. Our transplant nurse coordinator called today to arrange for our final crossmatch next week. Why do we have to repeat the crossmatch? We did it 3 months ago.

We repeat the crossmatch to be sure that you have not developed any antibodies to your sister's antigens. It is not always possible to identify a particular reason why the HLA antibodies are present, and they can appear and disappear from the serum quickly. Therefore it is necessary to perform a crossmatch close to the time of actual transplantation even if the crossmatch between a particular donor and recipient has been negative in the past. If you had an infection in the last 3 months or received a blood transfusion, you may have developed some new antibodies that may be directed against your sister's antigens. If you have developed antibodies toward your sister's antigens, you may reject her kidney after surgery.

PART FIVE

Surgery

How long will the kidney transplant
surgery take? How long will I be in the
hospital after my kidney transplant?

Where do they put my new kidney?
Do they remove my old kidneys when
I get my transplant?

How do they "hook up" my new kidney?

22. How long will the kidney transplant surgery take? How long will I be in the hospital after my kidney transplant?

Kidney transplant surgery takes 2 to 3 hours on average to perform. After surgery you will spend the night in the PACU (postanesthesia care unit) where you will be closely monitored. Your urine output is measured hourly and your IV (intravenous) fluids are adjusted hourly to match your urine output. You will have a tube in your bladder (Foley catheter) that drains your urine into a bag. This gives your bladder time to adapt to the new kidney and gives us a way to accurately measure your urine. The Foley catheter is usually removed on day 3 after surgery. The urine output is one measure of how your new kidney is working.

You will also notice a tube with a suction bulb on the end coming out near your new kidney. This is called a Jackson-Pratt drain. This drains fluids from your abdomen. It is removed a few days after surgery.

Most patients are in the hospital about 5 days after kidney transplant. This gives us time to give you the appropriate immunosuppressive medications and make sure your drug levels are acceptable. This also gives you time to familiarize yourself with your new medications. Your blood labs are drawn daily to assess your kidney function. Your urine output and fluid intake are closely monitored daily. You will be weighed daily. Your blood pressure, blood sugars, and vital signs are closely monitored. We are always looking for any signs of infection such as a fever or elevated white blood cell count.

Before you leave the hospital you should be out of bed and walking and familiar with your medications.

23. Where do they put my new kidney? Do they remove my old kidneys when I get my transplant?

The kidney transplant is placed in the iliac fossa (**Figure 1**). This is the area between your hip bone and pubic bone. Your native kidneys are located in a separate compartment. Your native kidneys are located in your back on either side of the spine below your lower ribs. When you get your transplant, your native kidneys typically atrophy (shrink).

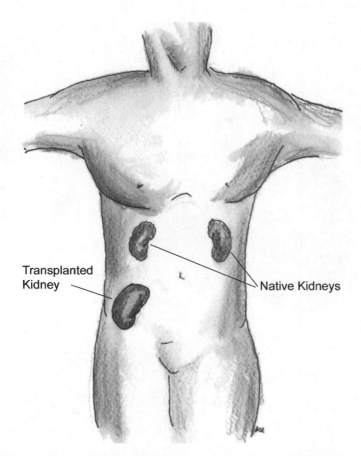

Figure 1   Where do they put my new kidney? Do they remove my old kidneys when I get my transplant?

Source: Courtesy of Dr. Khalid Khwaja.

24. How do they "hook up" my new kidney?

There are three "hook ups":

1. Renal artery
2. Renal vein
3. Ureter

The renal artery from your donor is sewn into your iliac artery (**Figure 2**). The renal vein from your donor kidney is sewn into the iliac vein. The ureter (the tube from the kidney to the bladder that carries the urine) from your donor is sewn into your bladder.

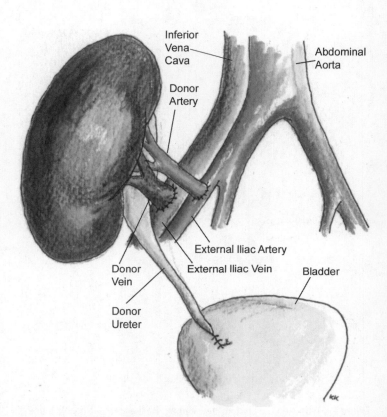

Figure 2   The renal artery from your donor is sewn into your iliac artery.

Source: Courtesy of Dr. Khalid Khwaja.

PART SIX

After Transplantation

How do you determine the amount
of immunosuppressive medications to
give to me?

How long will my kidney last?

What is the biggest challenge for the
future of kidney transplantation?

More . . .

25. My wife is coming home from the hospital tomorrow. She received a living donor kidney transplant from our daughter 5 days ago. She had a terrible time with dialysis, so we want this kidney to last. What can we do to ensure that the kidney will function for years to come?

One of the most important aspects of life after kidney transplant is the medication. The **immunosuppressive medications** are crucial to maintaining the kidney transplant. It is important that your wife becomes familiar with her immunosuppressive medications. The transplant nurse coordinator will educate your wife about these very important medications even before the surgery takes place. All medication instructions are carefully reviewed, including a schedule of when to take the medications. It's very helpful to set up a routine when you return home.

Immunosuppressive medications

Also referred to as antirejection medications, these drugs are prescribed to help your immune system accept your new organ and are taken for the rest of your life.

Many dialysis patients are in the habit of limiting their fluid intake. After kidney transplantation it is important to stay well hydrated. That means drinking enough fluid so that your intake of fluids is greater than your output of urine in a 24-hour period.

Your wife will be asked to monitor and record her vital signs (which includes weight, temperature, blood pressure, and heart rate) every day. Notify your transplant team immediately if your wife develops a temperature greater than 100.5°F. If there is a change in blood pressure or pulse, the transplant team should be contacted.

Your wife will have frequent blood labs to monitor her kidney function. In the first month after transplant, she will be seen by the transplant team weekly.

Initially after kidney transplantation your wife will notice a dramatic increase in her urine output. She will urinate frequently, often waking through the night to urinate. This is completely normal. Over time, her bladder will be able to hold a larger amount of urine so she will not have to urinate so frequently. If there is any burning or bleeding with urination, tell your transplant team about it. It may be related to a UTI (urinary tract infection). This can be easily tested for and treated with antibiotics.

Finally, it's important to use common sense! Good hand washing prevents the spread of infections. In the early days after surgery avoid people who are ill. Call the transplant team if you become ill.

26. How do you determine the amount of immunosuppressive medications to give to me?

You will receive sufficient immunosuppressive medication to maintain your kidney transplant but not so much that you develop infections.

In the operating room, you are given induction therapy. This is high-dose immunosuppressive medication that can include Solu-Medrol, Thymoglobulin, and mycophenolate. You receive these medications in the immediate days after your surgery and then you begin maintenance therapy. The maintenance therapy is mycophenolate and a calcineurin inhibitor or sirolimus. Some maintenance therapy includes prednisone. The maintenance therapy is the medication that you take at home. We are able to measure the levels of the calcineurin inhibitors and sirolimus. Studies have shown optimal levels for these medications.

27. How long will my kidney last?

The organ procurement and transplant network (OPTN) keeps statistics on graft survival. As of May 1, 2008, the

1-year adjusted survival for deceased donor non–expanded criteria donor kidney transplants was 91.7% for all ages of recipients. The 5-year survival was 70.4% and 10-year survival, 43.7%.

For expanded criteria donor kidney transplants, the 1-year adjusted graft survival was 84.8%, at 5 years 54.9%, and at 10 years 26.3%.

For living donor renal transplants, the adjusted graft survival at 1 year was 95.7%, at 5 years 80.8%, and at 10 years 57.9%. The adjusted survival rates above are an average across all age groups. There are many factors that affect the survival of kidney transplants, such as the original cause of the ESRD (end-stage renal disease), patient compliance, and living donor versus deceased donor.

28. What is the biggest challenge for the future of kidney transplantation?

First, finding donors is one of the biggest challenges for the future of kidney transplantation. The discrepancy between the number of patients on the waiting list and available donors is staggering. According to OPTN data from January 1, 2009, through September 30, 2009, there were 82,162 recipients waiting and only 7,923 deceased donors; live donation accounted for an additional 4,724 donors. Innovative ways to expand the live donor pool are being developed, such as paired and list exchanges and desensitization.

Second, most kidney transplant patients die of cardiovascular disease. We need to increase awareness about cardiovascular risk factors such as high cholesterol, diabetes mellitus, and hypertension and work harder to modify these risk factors.

The good news is that our understanding of the immune system has grown, and acute rejection has become a rare occurrence for our patients. More patients are being transplanted due to our ability to modify the immune response. Patients who would have been on the waiting list for years because of high antibody levels are being transplanted through processes such as desensitization.

After Transplantation

PART SEVEN

Complications

What is rejection? How do I know if I am rejecting my kidney transplant?

What else would make the serum creatinine rise abnormally?

29. What is rejection? How do I know if I am rejecting my kidney transplant?

Rejection occurs when your immune system attacks your kidney transplant. You receive the induction therapy and maintenance therapy so your body accepts your kidney transplant. This is called **engrafting**. Without immunosuppressive medications your immune system would recognize your transplant as a foreign invader and try to destroy it.

You will be closely followed after your transplant. We suspect rejection when your serum creatinine rises. Rejection is diagnosed on a tissue sample. We obtain the tissue sample by doing a kidney transplant biopsy. In a kidney transplant biopsy a small needle is inserted into your kidney transplant to remove a small piece of kidney. The tissue is examined under a microscope for signs of rejection. If rejection is present, there are medications that we can give you to halt the attack. In 2005 only 10% of patients who underwent kidney transplantation needed medication for rejection in their first year after surgery.

30. What else would make the serum creatinine rise abnormally?

Obstruction. When the serum creatinine rises, indicating a problem with the kidney, obstruction should always be ruled out. Obstruction is a blockage that usually affects the ureter and leads to increased pressure in the kidney (**Figure 3**). An abrupt decrease in urine output is a sign of obstruction. A renal transplant ultrasound can diagnose the obstruction and indicate where the problem is. The obstruction can be relieved

Rejection
When your immune system attacks your transplant.

Engrafting
The process of induction therapy and maintenance therapy so your body accepts your kidney transplant.

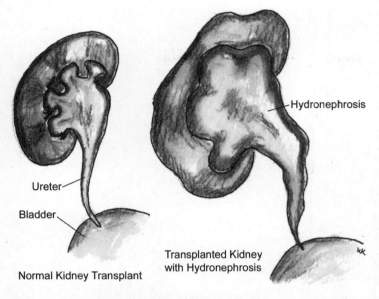

Figure 3   Obstruction is a blockage which usually affects the ureter and leads to increased pressure in the kidney.

Source: Courtesy of Dr. Khalid Khwaja.

by decompression. A tube can be put into the compressed area of the kidney or into the bladder. It is important to study the kidney, ureter, and bladder to determine the etiology of the obstruction. Obstruction is easily reversible.

Liver Transplantation

PART ONE

The Basics

What is the liver and why is it so important?

What are the complications of cirrhosis?

I have cirrhosis. At what point do I need to consider
a liver transplant?

More . . .

31. What is the liver and why is it so important?

The **liver** is the largest solid organ in the body. It is located on the right side of the abdomen (to the right of the stomach), behind the lower ribs and below the lungs. The liver is divided into two sections called lobes. In a healthy adult the liver is about the size of a football, weighing about 2.5 to 3 pounds. This organ receives its blood supply from two sources: the portal vein and the hepatic artery. The portal vein brings blood carrying nutrients to the liver from the intestine, and the hepatic artery brings blood and oxygen to the liver from the heart and lungs. The hepatic veins return blood to the heart (**Figure 4**). The liver performs more than 400 functions each day to keep the body healthy. Some of its major jobs are described here:

- Production of bile that permits the body to use protein, fat, and carbohydrates
- Use and storage of fats, sugars, iron, and vitamins
- Production of blood-clotting substances such as prothrombin
- Detoxification of drugs, alcohol, and other potentially harmful substances
- Production of a protein called albumin, which helps keep the body fluid within the blood vessels
- Monitoring for the presence of bacteria in the blood

32. What is cirrhosis?

Cirrhosis means severe scarring of the liver. When normal liver tissue is damaged, it changes into scar tissue or fibrosis. This scar tissue can reduce blood flow through the liver, making it difficult for the liver to carry out functions that are essential for life and health.

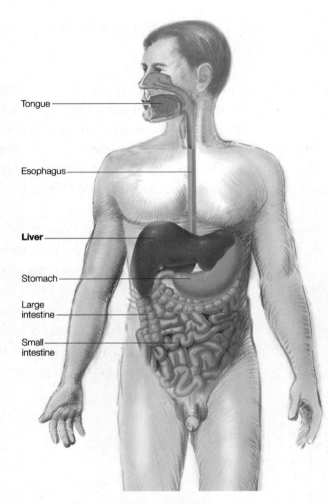

Tongue

Esophagus

Liver

Stomach

Large
intestine

Small
intestine

Figure 4   Location of the liver in the abdomen.

Many people believe that cirrhosis indicates a history of alcohol abuse, but this is not necessarily true. Many diseases and conditions may potentially cause severe scarring of the liver, including—but not limited to—alcohol abuse. A normal liver has no damage or scar tissue. As damage caused by disease progresses, liver cells die and turn into scar cells. Initially, only minimal scarring or fibrosis is present (stage 1). Fibrosis can advance to stage 2, then to stage 3, and ultimately to stage 4 or cirrhosis.

Cirrhosis rarely causes signs and symptoms in its early stages. When liver function deteriorates, fatigue, exhaustion, nausea, weight loss, and swelling in the legs and abdomen may occur. Jaundice—a yellowing of the skin and the whites of the eyes—and intense itching may develop as well. Cirrhosis has many causes (**Table 2**).

Alcohol is one of the most common causes of cirrhosis. It can directly injure healthy liver cells, so that these cells turn into scar tissue. Alcohol also brings damaging fat into the liver. In the United States alcohol is not the most common cause of cirrhosis. Fatty liver disease not associated with alcohol use, known as nonalcoholic steatohepatitis, is the leading cause of liver disease in this country. Infection with viruses such as hepatitis C

Table 2   Causes of Cirrhosis

Non-alcoholic steatohepatitis
Hepatitis C
Chronic hepatitis B
Alcoholic liver disease
Primary biliary cirrhosis
Primary sclerosing cholangitis
Hereditary hemochromatosis
Alpha-1 antitrypsin deficiency
Autoimmune hepatitis
Secondary biliary cirrhosis
Budd-Chiari syndrome
Wilson's disease
Congenital hepatic fibrosis
Biliary atresia
Cardiac failure
Cryptogenic cirrhosis

The Basics

(HCV) and hepatitis B (HBV) can also lead to cirrhosis. In addition, a number of inheritable conditions, such as hereditary hemochromatosis and alpha-1 antitrypsin deficiency, and autoimmune conditions, such as primary biliary cirrhosis and primary sclerosing cholangitis, can lead to cirrhosis.

33. What are the complications of cirrhosis?

Many people with cirrhosis have no signs or symptoms at all and feel quite well. In this condition, which is known as *compensated cirrhosis*, even though the liver is severely scarred, there are enough healthy cells within the scarred liver to perform all the necessary functions of a noncirrhotic liver. Most people with compensated cirrhosis remain in this condition for life and do not develop further complications of liver disease.

Over time, some people with compensated cirrhosis progress to *decompensated cirrhosis*. In this condition the liver is no longer capable of performing all its normal functions. Complications that people with decompensated cirrhosis may experience include bleeding varicose veins (varices) in the esophagus or stomach, accumulation of fluid in the abdomen (ascites), yellowing of the eyes and skin (jaundice), and confusion due to the liver's inability to clear toxins from the blood (hepatic encephalopathy).

34. What is portal hypertension?

To understand portal hypertension, one must first have a working knowledge of the normal blood flow into and out of the liver (**Figure 5**). Blood leaves the intestines and flows upward through the mesenteric veins to the portal vein. The blood in these vessels carries all

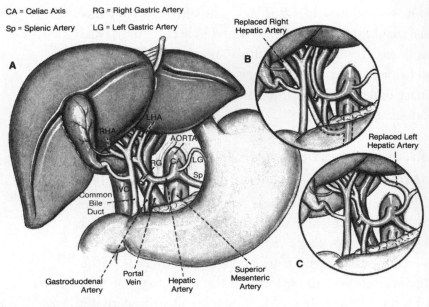

CA = Celiac Axis   RG = Right Gastric Artery

Sp = Splenic Artery   LG = Left Gastric Artery

Replaced Right
Hepatic Artery

A

B

LHA

RHA

AORTA

RG   CA   LG

Sp

Replaced Left
Hepatic Artery

VC

Common
Bile
Duct

Gastroduodenal
Artery

Portal
Vein

Hepatic
Artery

Superior
Mesenteric
Artery

C

Figure 5   Blood flow to the liver.

Source: Illustration courtesy of Roger Jenkins, MD, who holds the rights.

the nutrients and byproducts from digestion of food to the liver. Blood from the spleen also flows toward the portal vein, where it joins the blood from the mesenteric veins. The portal vein carries the blood into the liver and then splits into right and left branches. These branches then divide over and over again into small capillary vessels. A good analogy for this system is a tree: The tree trunk is the portal vein, and the large branches are the right and left portal veins. The twigs are the capillaries. A network of vessels also carries blood out of the liver to the heart. These vessels are called the hepatic veins.

To visualize how this system comes together, imagine two trees: one growing out of the ground (the portal vein system) and one hanging upside down from the sky (the hepatic vein system). The trees are connected together by their twigs. Blood flows through the liver by moving up the portal vein, traveling to the right or left branch, continuing on to the portal capillaries (twigs) and then into the hepatic vein capillaries (also twigs), up into the larger hepatic vein branches and ultimately into the inferior vena cava (the trunk of the upside-down tree). From there blood is carried to the heart.

When the liver is damaged due to cirrhosis, the blood finds it difficult to pass from the portal vein system into the hepatic vein system because the capillaries (twigs) are narrowed, twisted, and scarred. Nonetheless, blood continues to flow from the intestinal vessels and spleen toward the portal vein. This results in a "backup" of blood in the portal vein, causing high pressure there. High pressure in the portal vein is also known as **portal hypertension**.

Portal hypertension
When pressure in the portal vein becomes elevated, due to a damaged liver.

35. What is variceal bleeding?

One of the most significant complications of cirrhosis is variceal bleeding. It can occur if the pressure in the portal vein becomes elevated (portal hypertension). As mentioned in Question 34, blood enters the liver from the portal vein. When the liver is scarred, the blood flow through the liver can become restricted. Blood is a liquid and always tries to find the path of least resistance. This pathway may be around the liver rather than through the liver. In fact, one of the natural alternative routes circumventing the liver is through the vessels in the esophagus and stomach. These vessels typically carry a small amount of blood at low pressure. When the pressure in these vessels increases, they can rupture, causing a massive hemorrhage, vomiting of blood, and loss of consciousness.

The Basics

Variceal bleeding is treated with intravenous medications, with endoscopy, and later with pills called beta-blockers. More than 50% of patients awaiting liver transplantation have a variceal bleed before transplantation. Frequently, this bleeding is the initial event that prompts the primary gastroenterologist to refer the patient to a transplant center. Variceal bleeding is a dramatic event that continues to have a mortality rate of as much as 30% despite advances in therapy.

When patients are diagnosed with cirrhosis, endoscopic evaluation of the esophagus is necessary to assess for the presence of varices. During an endoscopy, the gastroenterologist administers intravenous sedation. The patient's throat is sprayed with a numbing medication to prevent gagging. An endoscope is then passed through the mouth and into the esophagus, stomach, and duodenum (first part of the small intestine). An endoscope is a long tube with a 1/4-inch caliber. On the end of the tube are a bright light and a tiny camera. The camera transmits video images to a television screen. Using this system the gastroenterologist can examine the inside of the esophagus and stomach to determine whether varices are present and, if so, whether they are large or small. If the patient has large varices, then beta-blockers can be started to significantly reduce the risk of variceal bleeding.

36. What is ascites, and why does it occur?

Ascites is a complication of portal hypertension and one of the most difficult complications to manage. As pressure builds in the portal vein, the body tries to reduce this pressure by leeching the liquid part of blood, called plasma, through the vessel walls into the abdomen. Although this transfer of plasma reduces portal pressure, it increases fluid accumulation in the body.

The management of ascites requires patience and close attention by both the physician and the patient. The initial treatment of ascites is restriction of dietary sodium to less than 2,000 milligrams per day and often fluid restriction to 2 liters per day. Diuretics can be added in a progressive, stepwise fashion.

37. Why do some people become confused or sleepy when they have cirrhosis?

Hepatic encephalopathy (HE) is a frequent but intermittent occurrence in many patients who are awaiting liver transplantation. One of the many jobs of the healthy liver is to clear toxins accumulated from food and metabolism from the bloodstream. When the amount of toxins produced exceeds the liver's ability to clear those toxins from the bloodstream, the person develops HE. This condition results in a temporary change in thought processing. Early signs of HE include insomnia and daytime sleepiness, difficulty concentrating on tasks, and forgetfulness. Later stages are characterized by irritability and other changes in personality, confusion, and sleeping most of the time. HE can even cause coma. This problem usually has an inciting cause, such as gastrointestinal bleeding, poor dietary habits, electrolyte abnormalities, renal failure, infection, and skipped or excessive medication. In patients presenting with HE, each of these potential causes must be considered and treatment should be directed at reversal of the particular cause.

The initial treatment of HE consists of lactulose. Lactulose is a sweet, syrupy liquid that absorbs toxins and causes diarrhea. It should be dosed so that the patient achieves three to five soft, controllable bowel movements per day. The antibiotics neomycin and rifaximin may be substituted for lactulose or added later if needed.

Many patients with HE are advised to avoid high protein intake. Of all the food types, protein causes much more toxin buildup as compared with fats and carbohydrates. Unfortunately, limiting the intake of protein may result in malnutrition, strength loss, and weight loss, increasing the risk of infection and a poor outcome after transplantation. Protein restriction should be reserved for only patients with HE that cannot be controlled in any other way.

38. I have cirrhosis. At what point do I need to consider a liver transplant?

The mere presence of cirrhosis is not an indication for liver transplantation. Many people with cirrhosis enjoy normal lives without ever developing complications or the need for hospitalization. Others decompensate over time, in which case transplantation may become necessary.

Patients often seek out a liver specialist when they first receive a diagnosis of cirrhosis in an effort to learn more about transplantation. Their initial hope may be to have a liver transplant—that is, to remove the damaged organ and replace it with a new, undamaged one. Although this outcome might, on the surface, seem to be a good solution, several negative factors must be considered before pursuing this option. First, the rate of surgical complications of liver transplantation may be as high as 15% to 20%, including death within the first year after transplantation. You must weigh this risk against the risk of death without transplantation, taking into account quality of life issues. Second, the medications required after transplantation have many side effects. Early exposure to these medications may result in a diminished quality of life for at least some time after the operation. Third, organ availability is limited in many regions of the country. As a consequence the degree of illness necessary to be at the top of the transplant waiting list can be quite high. Patients with compensated cirrhosis will likely remain at the lower end of the waiting list for a long time.

Patients should consider liver transplantation when they have developed complications of liver disease such as ascites, variceal bleeding, hepatic encephalopathy, or jaundice (**Table 3**). Additionally, even in patients who feel well, a rising MELD score (see Question 46) may be an indication for transplant evaluation. The development of liver cancer may also be an indication for transplantation. Careful monitoring by a physician is necessary in all patients with cirrhosis to look for signs of liver failure so that referral for transplantation occurs at the appropriate time.

The progression of liver disease is often predictable. Most patients with cirrhosis have already developed complications of liver disease such as ascites, variceal bleeding, jaundice, or encephalopathy. These symptoms may come and go, and the patient may sometimes feel quite well. This is an ideal time for liver

Table 3   Complications of Cirrhosis

Jaundice
Ascites
Variceal Bleeding
Hepatic Encephalopathy
Malnutrition
Edema
Poor protein production
Poor clotting factor production

transplantation. Unfortunately, because of the system of organ distribution, we rarely have the opportunity to offer liver transplantation at the most opportune time. Livers are distributed according to the MELD scoring system (see Question 46). The MELD scoring system prioritizes patient who are "sicker" based on their laboratory tests (bilirubin, INR, and creatinine). These lab tests may not, however, reflect the true degree of illness in some people, especially those with ascites, bleeding problems, and malnutrition. This situation may lead to a seesaw of emotions—the desire to rise to the top of the list requires increased illness, but this is a condition no one wishes to achieve.

On rare occasions candidates for liver transplantation may become "too sick" to undergo transplantation. This situation occurs most commonly when the candidate develops infection or sepsis. In such a case the infection is often caused by bacteria that enter the urinary bladder, kidneys, ascites fluid, lungs (pneumonia), or bloodstream. Sepsis can lead to failure of organs other than the liver, such as the kidneys, lungs, heart, and blood vessel (vascular) system. When patients have sepsis, liver transplantation cannot be performed for several reasons:

- Immunosuppressive agents are required after transplantation, but they limit the body's ability to assist in fighting off the infection.
- The patient's blood pressure may be too low to safely perform surgery.
- The patient's blood pressure may be too low to adequately supply the new liver with blood.
- If other organs are in failure, a liver transplant may not help the patient achieve total recovery.

In this circumstance it is better to attempt to control the infection and then proceed to transplantation, rather than the reverse. Unfortunately, when sepsis is present and the liver is not functioning properly, it is difficult for the body to recover adequately to allow later transplantation. It is therefore important to report all signs of infection to your doctor so that early treatment can be initiated and sepsis prevented.

The Basics

PART TWO

Before Transplantation

Who is a candidate for liver transplantation?

What questions should I ask my transplant team to make sure I have chosen the best one for me?

What about patients with liver cancer?

More . . .

39. Who is a candidate for liver transplantation?

If you have cirrhosis with at least some degree of decompensation, you may be a candidate for liver transplantation. To qualify as a candidate for a liver transplant, you must be healthy enough to undergo surgery, be reliable with medication and follow-up appointments, and have a support system at home to help you with your post-transplant program.

Some problems may disqualify you from receiving a liver transplant:

• Alcohol or other substance abuse within at least 6 months before consideration for placement on the waiting list
• Metastatic (spreading) malignancy of the liver or other types of cancer
• Other serious diseases, such as uncontrolled infections, uncorrectable heart disease, or severe lung disease
• A history of missing your appointments and poor adherence to or noncompliance with prescribed medications
• Inadequate support from family or friends
• Human immunodeficiency virus (HIV)-positive status
• A history of multiple upper abdominal surgeries
• Advanced age
• Morbid obesity

Alcoholism is one of the most common causes of liver disease both in the United States and worldwide. Today, alcoholic liver disease is second only to hepatitis C as an indication for transplantation. Many years ago there were debates about whether patients with liver dysfunction due to alcoholic liver disease qualified for transplantation. Since then, our understanding of alcoholism has evolved; it is now viewed as a disease and, as such, patients suffering from alcoholism receive access equal to that of nonalcoholics in terms of transplants.

The vast majority (more than 90%) of the transplant programs in the United States require at least 6 months of total sobriety before transplantation may be considered. The reasoning behind this requirement is neither punishment nor an intentional delay in placement of patients with alcoholic liver disease on the waiting list. Rather, the liver, as a regenerative organ, can improve with abstinence to the point where liver transplantation may no longer be necessary. This process of functional regeneration continues for 1 year or more after stopping alcohol use but is most dramatic during the first 6 months of abstinence. If the patient continues to show signs of liver failure and portal hypertensive complications after 6 months of abstinence, the likelihood of recovery to normal liver function is low, and transplantation may be necessary. Most programs also require the patient to undergo rehabilitation and counseling during this 6-month time frame.

The success rates of liver transplantation for alcoholic liver disease are equal to the results for transplantation in cases of nonalcoholic disease. In fact, for those who remain abstinent from alcohol after transplantation, the long-term results may even be better because recurrent disease (such as hepatitis C) is not a concern.

40. What questions should I ask my transplant team to make sure I have chosen the best one for me?

You should ask the following questions to a member of the transplant team:

1. Are there any other options besides transplantation?
2. What are the risks and benefits of transplantation?

3. Tell me about the evaluation process.

4. Where is the transplant evaluation performed?

5. How will I know if I am on the transplant waiting list?

6. How long do most patients with my blood type wait for transplantation in this region?

7. How long have this hospital and team been doing liver transplants?

8. Who are the transplant team members?

9. What are the organ and patient survival rates at 1, 3, and 5 years at this hospital?

10. Will I be given an expanded criteria donor organ? How is that decision made?

11. Does this program offer living donor transplantation? How many of these procedures have been done so far?

12. How many surgeons will operate on me? How many are attending physicians, fellows, and residents?

13. Is there a special unit in the hospital for transplant recipients?

14. Whom can I call with questions about the transplant process?

15. Will I be asked to participate in research studies?

16. Can I tour the transplant center facility and hospital transplant floor?

41. What is a cadaver liver?

A cadaver (or deceased donor) liver is an organ obtained from a brain-dead donor to be used for liver transplantation. In the unfortunate circumstance of a previously healthy person's death, his or her family may choose to give the "gift of life" and donate the deceased person's organs. Until 1998 cadavers were the only adult liver donors in the United States. More recently, organs have been obtained from healthy living donors—hence the need to distinguish between deceased liver donors and live liver donors.

Most organ donors are people who suffer from head injuries that result in brain death. These head injuries may include a stroke, trauma after a car accident or fall, or brain tumor that has not metastasized. Death can be declared in two ways in such cases: when a person's heart stops beating (cardiac death) or when the person's brain ceases to function (brain death). Brain death occurs when blood and oxygen cannot flow to the brain, even though the heart is still beating and providing blood and oxygen to other parts of the body. Patients with brain death usually require a ventilator or breathing machine to bring oxygen into the lungs. In brain death the organs remain functional and can be used for transplantation after a physician declares the patient to be brain dead. Because of the potential for conflict of interest, this physician may not be part of a transplant team.

Anyone up to 85 years of age may be eligible to donate organs and/or tissue. If it becomes appropriate to evaluate someone for organ and/or tissue donation, a trained coordinator reviews the person's medical history to determine if he or she can be a donor. People who have died by brain death may be able to donate all of their organs and tissue.

It is important to discuss the issue of organ donation with your family members and your next-of-kin. In most states merely identifying yourself as an organ donor on your driver's license does not automatically result in organ donation; the surviving family must agree to donation as well. Organ donors are treated the same way as nonorgan donors in emergency situations, so you do not have to fear that identification as an organ donor would result in inferior medical care. The donor's body is not disfigured, so an open-casket funeral can still be an option. There is no charge for being an organ donor.

On rare occasions a friend or family member of a transplant candidate may die during the waiting period. If the deceased becomes brain-dead and his or her family wishes to donate the organs, they may choose **directed donation**. This means that the donated organs can be directed specifically to the transplant candidate. The MELD score becomes irrelevant in such a case, and the candidate receives the liver as long as there is an acceptable blood type and size match. The other organs may also be directly donated or go into the standard organ transplant matching system.

42. I am the provider in my family and don't usually ask for help. Do I need anyone to help me get through this process?

Liver transplantation requires a major commitment from not only the recipient but also that person's family and support network. An individual often takes many things for granted before becoming ill with liver disease—for example, going to work, driving a car, pushing a grocery cart in the supermarket, and taking medications. After the need for transplantation has been identified, many of these tasks can be difficult to accomplish alone due to weakness, fatigue, and the side effects of medications. Immediately after transplantation, you will not have enough strength or stamina to carry out routine tasks for several months and will need help. Your friends and family must be available to drive

---

Directed donation

Donated organs can be directed specifically to a transplant candidate on the rare occasion that a friend or family member of a transplant candidate may die during the waiting period. If the deceased becomes brain-dead, his or her family may choose this option.

you to and from your doctors' appointments, to provide food and medications, and to watch for complications of the transplant surgery. You will not likely need 24 hour a day nursing care or observation. In fact, you will be able to move freely around your home and gradually go out for short periods of time. Your reliance on others will not last forever; usually, transplant recipients regain their independence in 3 to 6 months.

43. What about patients with liver cancer?

Liver cancer is a feared complication of cirrhosis. For patients with cirrhosis on the waiting list, the risk of developing liver cancer can range from 1% to 10%. Transplant physicians periodically test the liver for the development of liver cancer by performing an alpha-fetoprotein (AFP) blood test and conducting an ultrasound, CT (computed tomography), or MRI (magnetic resonance imaging) of the liver.

Some, but not all, patients with liver cancer may be candidates for liver transplantation. To be a viable candidate, the patient must fit into the **Milan Criteria** (developed in Milan, Italy). The Milan Criteria state that the patient with liver cancer has a low risk of recurrence after transplantation if

1. There is a single tumor measuring less than or equal to 5 centimeters in diameter, or
2. There are two or three tumors, each measuring less than 3 centimeters in diameter (**Figure 6**).

In each case there must be no evidence that the tumor has spread outside the liver or into blood vessels. A CT or MRI of the abdomen and chest and other tests as needed can rule out spread of the tumor. If there are

Milan Criteria

Criteria to select patients with liver cancer to be viable candidates for transplantation. The Milan Criteria state that the patient with liver cancer has a low risk of recurrence after transplantation if there is a single tumor measuring less than or equal to 5 centimeters in diameter, or there are two or three tumors, each measuring less than 3 centimeters in diameter.

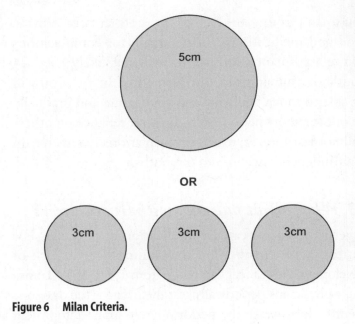

Figure 6   Milan Criteria.

four tumors in the liver, regardless of their size, the patient is characterized as "outside Milan Criteria."

In the past, before the Milan Criteria were established and applied, liver transplantation was attempted for a variety of tumor sizes and numbers. When transplantation occurred "outside Milan Criteria," the likelihood of a tumor recurring in the newly transplanted liver was nearly 80% within 1 year and nearly 100% within 3 years. The reason the tumor is thought to recur in the transplanted liver is related to immunosuppression. The intact immune system has the ability to identify and eradicate any stray tumor cells that may have escaped the liver. Once the liver transplant is performed and the patient begins to take immunosuppressive drugs, however, the immune system may lose its ability to recognize and kill these cells. The tumor cells may then return to the new liver or settle in other sites, such as the lungs or bones.

Unfortunately, chemotherapy either before or after transplantation has been largely ineffective in changing the tumor recurrence rates.

Some patients with liver cancer may be candidates for surgical resection of the tumor while awaiting liver transplantation. This procedure may be an option only for patients who have good liver function, minimal ascites, and a tumor located in the left lobe or lower periphery of the right lobe. Other candidates may be treated with radiofrequency ablation (RFA), transarterial chemoembolization (TACE), or with transarterial radioactive beads in an effort to control the growth of the tumor to remain within the Milan Criteria while awaiting transplantation.

44. Who pays for the transplant?

Financial planning is an important part of the transplant process. Each transplant program includes a financial coordinator to help you understand the cost of transplantation, your insurance transplant benefits, and the overall financial process. You need to know how much your insurance will pay not only for the transplant itself but also for medications after the transplant takes place. You may find it necessary to draw on savings accounts, investments, federal and private assistance options, and fundraising. The financial coordinator and a social worker can answer questions about insurance coverage and assist you in identifying financial resources available to you.

During your evaluation, you will meet with the social worker and the financial coordinator to discuss financial and social issues in detail. Some insurance companies require a review of your evaluation results to determine whether you meet their criteria before they will agree to pay for a transplant. If you are a good candidate for a transplant, the transplant program works with you in obtaining insurance approval from your insurance company. Gaining insurance approval is ultimately the patient's responsibility, however.

The cost of transplantation and follow-up varies across the United States. You must consider many potential costs—some directly related to your medical care and others that are unrelated to the surgery. Direct medical care costs include pretransplant evaluation and testing; surgery and the postoperative hospital stay; subsequent hospital stays for complications; outpatient follow-up care and testing; antirejection, and other drugs; fees for the hepatologist, surgeon, and anesthesiologist; physical therapy and rehabilitation; and insurance deductibles and copayments. Indirect costs include transportation to and from the transplant center, food and lodging for your family, child care, and lost wages for you and some family members.

Few patients are able to pay for all costs of transplantation from a single income source. Although health insurance companies cover many of the direct costs, savings accounts and other private funds will likely be necessary to pay for other expenses. The transplant social worker and the financial coordinator may be able to suggest alternative sources of funding for those in need, such as charitable organizations, fundraisers, and advocacy groups.

If you *have* insurance coverage:

- Transplants are very expensive, so you should make sure your healthcare policy does not include any special riders or limitations pertaining to such procedures.

Prescription coverage is imperative, as the costs of transplant medications are high. If you have a health maintenance organization (HMO) or point of service (POS) insurance plan, make sure you obtain all necessary referrals to avoid any billing issues.

• If your health plan covers only partial costs, your social worker and/or financial coordinator can help you find ways to finance the out-of-pocket expenses. There are programs designed to assist transplant recipients with their unique financial needs.

If you *do not have* health insurance coverage:

• Not having health insurance poses a challenge for patients in need of transplants, but your financial coordinator can help you investigate other options, such as state or federal funding or insurance and assistance through charitable organizations or advocacy groups.

• Check with your local Medicaid office to see whether you are eligible for this coverage, which is based primarily on income. In addition, most states operate a high-risk health insurance pool for individuals with preexisting conditions who need to purchase an insurance plan. Check with your state's insurance commissioner for more information.

• On the Internet, you can log on to your state's website to find links to government agencies dealing with insurance or health care. You can also consult your local phone book for agency listings under the government section.

• Several agencies will assist you in fundraising, and the social worker and financial coordinator can provide you with information on these resources. If you are out of work due to disability, you should apply for Social Security Disability Insurance. You will become eligible for Medicare coverage after receiving these Social Security benefits for 2 years. For more information, consult the websites for Medicare or the Centers for Medicare and Medicaid Services.

45. What is a liver transplant evaluation?

People who have a diseased liver may consider transplantation as a treatment option. A transplant evaluation is necessary to determine the risks and benefits of transplantation for each individual, identify potential problems, discuss the options of a living donor transplant, and identify risks for the potential donor.

Much of your transplant-related care will be handled by a transplant hepatologist—a medical physician with expertise in liver disease and management of patients with cirrhosis awaiting liver transplantation. Additional consultation with a cardiologist for people with heart disease, a pulmonologist for patients with lung problems, a nephrologist for candidates with kidney problems, and an endocrinologist for patients with diabetes may be ordered as needed.

The evaluation for transplantation usually takes place on an outpatient basis but may occur when you are an inpatient in urgent circumstances. During the evaluation you will have a number of medical tests:

• Blood tests to determine your blood type, liver and kidney function, and viruses to which you may have been exposed in the past, such as hepatitis A, B, and C and HIV
• A chest x-ray to see if your lungs are healthy
• A Doppler ultrasound and/or MRI of the liver, which enables the physician to see your liver and the flow of blood through the arteries and veins

- Tuberculosis testing, called a PPD skin test
- An electrocardiogram (ECG)

You may also be asked to undergo additional tests such as a colonoscopy, upper endoscopy, echocardiogram, cardiac stress test, and lung function tests.

If you are being evaluated for liver transplantation, you will see a number of healthcare professionals who can assess these issues:

- A transplant surgeon will discuss the operation.
- A social worker will help you identify some of the issues you are facing and talk with you about your ability to handle the responsibilities that come with being a transplant recipient.
- An infectious disease doctor will identify any active or potential issues with infection.
- A psychiatrist, along with the social worker, will help you identify and handle troubling issues such as depression.
- A financial coordinator, along with the social worker, will help you understand insurance issues about liver transplant.
- A nutritionist will help you plan a diet that will keep you in the best possible health.

You will also meet with a transplant nurse coordinator. The coordinator is an important person in your care— he or she acts as a liaison between you and the other healthcare providers. You can view the coordinator as a resource for information at all points along your path to transplantation.

After your transplant evaluation is complete, the transplant team reviews all the information gathered in this process.

The team may make recommendations for other necessary tests and vaccinations. Ultimately, the team members decide whether it is the appropriate time to list you for liver transplantation, whether there are outstanding issues that need attention, or whether you are not a candidate for transplantation. A member of the transplant team will see you at a follow-up appointment in the office to discuss this decision and its impact on your future health care.

PART THREE

Organ Allocation

What is the MELD score and how does it work?

Where will my liver come from?

Can I be evaluated and listed at more than one program? Do I have to move there?

More . . .

46. What is the MELD score and how does it work?

The Model for End-stage Liver Disease (MELD) score was developed in 1994 to assess the risk of a procedure called transjugular portosystemic shunt. Later, the **MELD score** was evaluated as a tool to rank patients on the liver transplant waiting list and found to be a fair way to assign cadaveric organs to those most in need of transplantation. The MELD score is actually a question that is answered by a mathematical calculation (**Table 4**): "What is the risk of dying with liver disease in the next 3 months?" In essence, it is a crystal ball with ability to look 3 months into the future. Its accuracy is quite good but, of course, not perfect.

To calculate the MELD score three laboratory tests are necessary: the total bilirubin level, the international normalized ratio (INR), and the creatinine level. Inserting these laboratory values into the MELD formula yields a score between 6 and 40. As shown in Table 4 a score of 6 indicates a 1% chance of dying during the next 3 months and therefore the need for liver transplantation is very small. A MELD score of

MELD score

A tool to rank patients on the liver transplant waiting list to assign cadaveric organs to those most in need of transplantation. The MELD score is actually a question that is answered by a mathematical calculation: "What is the risk of dying with liver disease in the next 3 months?"

Table 4   MELD Score Mortality Equivalents

6	1%
22	10%
24	15%
26	20%
29	30%
31	40%
33	50%
35	60%
37	70%
38	80%
40	90%

40 means there is a 90% chance of death in the next 3 months and transplantation is urgently needed.

The MELD scoring system has been extensively evaluated by the transplant community and is believed to be fair, objective, and unbiased. The MELD score and ranking for liver transplantation do not take into account subjective elements such as quality of life, ability to work, degree of pain, length of time on the waiting list, and number of hospitalizations. In fact, even liver-related complications such as variceal bleeding, ascites, and encephalopathy are not considered in the score. Before the MELD scoring system was approved for ranking candidates on the liver transplant waiting list, it was extensively researched and a computer model was developed based on the experiences of actual patients. The MELD system places all its emphasis on the candidate's *risk of death* rather than on his or her quality of life. Compared with the previous ranking system, the MELD system is more effective in preventing death before transplantation. Patients are now more likely to have an opportunity to have life-saving transplantation rather than waiting while the less ill undergo transplantation.

The liver transplant waiting list is actually four lists, separated by blood type: O, A, B, and AB. Within each list patients are prioritized by their MELD scores. When a donor liver becomes available, it is matched with the candidate on the waiting list with the highest MELD score in the identical blood group. A person with a MELD score of 29 is ranked ahead of a person with a MELD score of 25. If the donor is a child, the liver is matched with the highest-ranking pediatric recipient.

The MELD score can be reassessed as often as the patient's physician believes it is necessary. Any updated information can be used to recalculate and therefore rerank patients on the waiting list. For patients with a MELD score in the range of 6 to 10, new MELD scores must be assessed at least once per year. For scores between 10 and 18, updates every 6 months are necessary. For scores between 18 and 24, new lab data are necessary every month. Scores over 24 require weekly updates.

The UNOS system divides the United States into 11 regions (**Figure 7**). Organs are procured and distributed within each region. For example, a blood type A liver donated in region 1 goes to the highest-ranking candidate on the blood type A list in region 1. Because of this regional procurement and distribution of organs, each region has its own supply and demand for livers. Regions with a high supply of donor organs and a

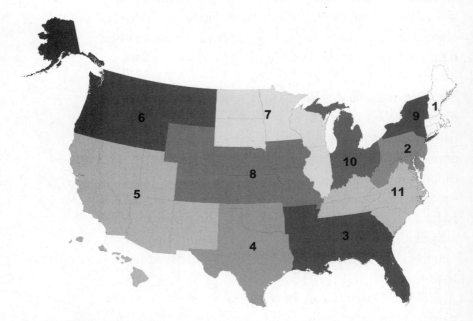

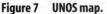

Figure 7   UNOS map.

small demand are able to transplant candidates with lower MELD scores than regions with low supplies and high demands. This often results in regional inequities in the MELD score needed to appear at the top of the waiting list.

Your position on the waiting list is based exclusively on your MELD score. Movement up (and down) the list is determined by changes in your bilirubin, INR, and creatinine. In the past the amount of time spent waiting on the list was an important factor in your position on the list. Now waiting time is not considered when determining your rank. For this reason your doctors may choose to watch you and follow the progression of your liver disease before listing you for transplantation. The transplant team is aware of the typical score required in each region for transplantation and can evaluate and possibly list you as your score approaches the top of the waiting list.

There are presently no limitations on the number and locations of transplant centers you can be evaluated by and listed with. If you and your doctors believe that your condition would benefit from transplantation earlier than might be provided in your home region, you may seek out transplantation in a region that provides organs to patients with lower MELD scores. Unfortunately, there are numerous drawbacks to evaluation and listing outside your home region: fewer readily available family and friend support systems; necessity to travel for evaluation, transplantation, and frequent office visits; and insurance plans that may not cover out-of-region transplantation expenses.

Another option if you seek to undergo transplantation with a low MELD score may be living donor liver transplantation (discussed in Part 4).

Primary graft nonfunction (PGNF)

A condition that occurs within 1 week after organ transplantation. PGNF is not caused by rejection or blocked blood vessels; some transplanted organs do not work properly after surgery. These patients are usually in critical condition and experience organ failure within 48 hours after transplantation; they require immediate retransplantation and take priority over the MELD scoring system to receive the next available organ from an acceptable blood type–matched donor.

Fulminant hepatic failure

A condition whereby a toxin (e.g., acetaminophen toxicity, mushroom poisoning) or virus (e.g., hepatitis A or hepatitis B) affects a previously healthy person with a normal liver. The risk of death from this condition is extremely high, and these patients take priority over the MELD scoring system to receive the next available liver from an acceptable blood type–matched donor.

Status 1 is a special designation for patients with fulminant hepatic failure and **primary graft nonfunction (PGNF)**. The risk of death from these two conditions is extremely high. Status 1 patients take priority over the MELD scoring system so that these patients can receive the next available liver from an acceptable blood type–matched donor. In this circumstance patients may receive an identically blood type–matched or a blood type O (universal donor) liver.

Fulminant hepatic failure occurs when a toxin or virus affects a previously healthy person with a normal liver. Examples include acetaminophen toxicity, mushroom poisoning, and rare instances of hepatitis A or hepatitis B. Affected individuals develop jaundice (yellowing of the eyes and skin) followed within 8 weeks by hepatic encephalopathy (confusion caused by the liver's inability to clear toxins from the blood).

PGNF occurs within 1-2 weeks after liver transplantation. Rarely and for unclear reasons, do some transplanted livers not work properly after surgery. PGNF is not caused by rejection or blocked blood vessels. These patients are usually in critical condition and experience liver failure within 48 hours after transplantation; they require immediate retransplantation.

There is no way to predict how long it takes to move to the top of the transplant waiting list. Because the list is organized by blood group and MELD score, waiting time is no longer relevant in distributing donor organs. Until February 2002, when the MELD scoring system was implemented, waiting time was a critical factor in getting to the top of the list. Simply put, the longer you were on the list, the higher on the list you were placed. The list worked very much like a line to buy movie tickets: If you waited long enough, eventually you got to the ticket window. Because this system allowed people who were not in desperate need to undergo transplantation while terribly ill patients died without the opportunity to receive a donor organ, it was abandoned. Additionally, the candidate's location on the list depended more on when the referring physician decided to send the patient to the transplant program than on the patient's actual degree of illness.

The MELD system is based exclusively on the degree of illness and risk of death before transplantation. Waiting time cannot be predicted because receipt of an organ requires deterioration in health, especially in the three critical lab tests: total bilirubin, INR, and creatinine. Primary care physicians, gastroenterologists, and transplant physicians work diligently with their patients to keep them healthy. The goal is to keep patients well enough so that transplantation is a last resort.

Certain UNOS regions in the United States have larger supplies and fewer demands for livers than other regions. The result is variations in waiting times across the country. When the demand is high and the supply of donor livers is low, a person must have a higher MELD score to appear at the top of the list. The score needed to undergo transplantation in such regions is often in the range of 30 to 35. Other regions have large numbers of liver donors, so transplantation can occur at lower MELD scores in the 18 to 20 range. The reasons for the regional differences in donation rates are not clear but may include differences in fatality rates from motor vehicle crashes, access to major hospitals, regional customs and beliefs, and expertise of organ banks in recruiting donors.

47. Where will my liver come from?

UNOS divides the United States into 11 regions for organ distribution purposes (see Figure 7). Patients waiting for liver transplantation in a specific region most likely get a liver from their own region, typically from the local organ procurement organization (OPO). An OPO is an organization that is accepted as a member of the OPTN and is authorized by the Centers for Medicare and Medicaid Services (CMS) to procure organs for transplantation. Each OPO has a defined geographic procurement territory within which the organization concentrates its procurement efforts. A region can have one or more OPOs providing organ procurement services to various locations in the region.

When a deceased donor liver becomes available, a standardized protocol is followed to place the organ in the proper candidate on the waiting list. The liver waiting list emphasizes the degree of illness but also incorporates the locations of the donor and the recipient. Status 1 patients have the highest priority for the donor liver first within the local (OPO) territory and then within the region. If there are no status 1 candidates on the regional list, the liver goes to the candidate with the highest MELD score above 15 within the local area. If no candidates satisfy this criterion, then the liver stays within the region and goes to the person with the highest MELD score above 15. If no candidates in the region have a MELD score greater than 15, then the liver goes to the person with the highest MELD score first in the local area and then in the region. If there are still no appropriate recipients, the liver is offered to a status 1 patient outside the donor's region. This system ensures that the sickest local/regional patient has the best opportunity to undergo liver transplantation.

48. Can my new liver give me any illnesses? Is it tested for HIV before I get it?

The organ bank tests donor organs extensively before their transplantation. Tests for infection with human immunodeficiency virus (HIV), hepatitis B virus, and hepatitis C virus are performed, and the information is given to the transplant team. Depending on the recipient's disease and severity of illness, the transplant team has the option of using organs with known infections. Many research studies have shown that placing a donor liver with hepatitis C into a recipient with hepatitis C is safe and does not confer any excess risk of liver failure or severity of recurrent hepatitis C. Similarly, patients with hepatitis B can be transplanted with organs from donors with hepatitis B. HIV-positive organs are not used, however.

Livers are tested not only for viruses but also other infections and conditions that might potentially be passed on to the recipient. For example, a donor with a severe blood infection with the *Staphylococcus* bacteria may not be considered a safe donor because the bacterial infection would likely be transmitted to the recipient. Even if the recipient is currently taking preventive antibiotics, he or she will soon be immunosuppressed; as a consequence, the risk of overwhelming infection immediately after transplantation is very high. The liver and other abdominal organs are also inspected for the presence of non–liver-related cancer.

Organ banks are also adept at acquiring historical information about the donor. Important factors in determining the donor's eligibility include the donor's history of drug use, sexual contact, home situation, nutrition, and prior cancers such as melanoma, basal cell skin cancer, and breast cancer. These considerations are risk factors for the potential presence of infectious diseases and communicable malignancies. This information, when provided to the recipient's transplant team, can be used in making the decision whether to accept that particular organ for the recipient.

49. Can I be evaluated and listed at more than one program? Do I have to move there?

Liver transplantation candidates can be listed at more than one center at any given time but do not benefit from being listed by two programs within the same organ allocation region. All transplant programs within a UNOS region work from the same master list.

If a patient chooses to be listed by two programs, he or she should be evaluated in different UNOS regions to minimize the waiting time. It is not a UNOS requirement that patients move their homes to the transplant center's region. However, you must consider some additional issues when seeking a multiple listing. First, your health insurance company may not pay for a transplant at a center outside of your local region. Second, if the insurer does agree to pay for the transplant wherever it occurs first, the payer often will not cover the expenses of transportation and accommodation for you and your family. Third, organs become available on very short notice, and you must be able to get to the transplant center quickly once the organ is ready. Fourth, most programs require their recipients to remain in close proximity to the transplant center for a month or more after the operation to monitor the recovery, watch for rejection, and adjust medications as needed. Finally, if serious posttransplant complications arise, you must be prepared to return to the transplant center for care. These requirements can be very expensive and time-consuming for both patient and family. Even though the waiting time may be shorter at a particular center outside of your home region, it may not be the best overall plan to be transplanted there.

PART FOUR

Live Donor Liver Transplantation

What is a live donor liver transplant?

Who can be a live liver donor? What are the risks?

Are the results as good if I have a living donor compared with a cadaver donor?

50. What is a live donor liver transplant?

The unique anatomy of the liver allows it to be separated into independent anatomic units that are able to retain their normal function (**Figure 8**). Since 1989 several thousand **live donor liver transplant (LDLT)** operations have been performed worldwide, most commonly between an adult donor and a pediatric recipient. These procedures have significantly reduced

Live donor liver transplant (LDLT)

In these highly technical operations, the right lobe of the donor's liver (about 60% of the total liver) is implanted into the recipient. The recipient's entire liver is removed because it is diseased and functions poorly. After surgery, the rapid regeneration of the liver allows both the donor's and the recipient's livers to return to nearly full size.

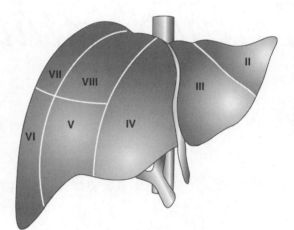

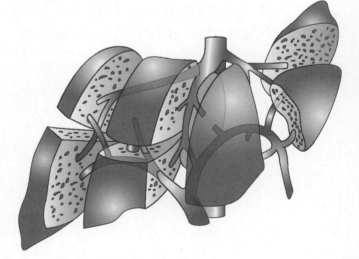

Figure 8   Liver segments.

Source: Reprinted with permission from Memorial Sloan-Kettering.

the number of pediatric patients who die while on the waiting list.

Current data suggest that the results of live donor liver transplants are at least similar to, and perhaps better than, the results of deceased donor liver transplants. Because it can potentially increase the number of people who may benefit from liver transplantation, LDLT poses exciting, new surgical possibilities for adult patients with end-stage liver disease. The basis for taking part of a living person's liver lies in a healthy liver's unique ability to grow back or regenerate to normal size for both the donor and the recipient.

In these highly technical operations, the right lobe of the donor's liver (about 60% of the total liver) is implanted into the recipient. The recipient's entire liver is removed because it is diseased and functions poorly. After surgery, the rapid regeneration of the liver allows both the donor's and the recipient's livers to return to nearly full size. Amazingly, it typically takes the recipient's liver less than 1 month to regenerate fully. That time frame is a bit longer for the donor, whose liver often takes a full year to accomplish the same feat.

Because the left lobe is the smaller of the two lobes, it can be used as a living donor organ only in children or very small adults. The larger right lobe is needed when the recipient is an average-size or larger adult.

51. Who can be a live liver donor? What are the risks?

A potential donor must first volunteer to donate a portion of his or her liver to a family member or someone with whom he or she shares strong emotional ties. Not all volunteers, however, are deemed suitable. The donor's blood type must be compatible with the recipient's blood type (see Table 6), and his or her liver must be large enough relative to the recipient's body size. Many live donor transplant centers also enforce age and weight limitations. Typically, donors must be at least 18 years of age. This not only increases the likelihood of an adequate donor liver size but also ensures that the donor is of legal age to consent to the procedure. It would certainly be awkward—if not unethical—for a cirrhotic parent to consent to both his or her own operation and the donor's operation. Careful screening tests must be performed to evaluate the health and suitability of the donor. These tests include basic laboratory tests, a full medical evaluation, and imaging (CT or MRI) of the liver to determine the size of each lobe and the vascular (blood vessel) anatomy.

The decision to donate part of one's liver can be extremely difficult. By definition, the donor is healthy and, therefore, does not need major abdominal surgery and its attendant risks. Many factors must be considered in this decision, including the medical issues mentioned previously. Does the donor have something to gain from the operation—specifically, more quality time with the healthy recipient? How would the donor feel about the surgery if he or she developed a complication? What about if the recipient had a complication or died? Psychiatric evaluations are conducted to ensure that the donor does not feel unduly pressured by other family members and is truly willing to undergo the procedure.

As with any surgical procedure, there are risks involved in donating a part of the liver. Living donors receive general anesthesia for the operation, and live donor liver transplantation is considered major surgery. All patients experience some discomfort and pain after an operation. Living donors may develop complications such as infections, bleeding, or even death.

Although most donors report an overall positive experience, it is possible to have negative psychological consequences from such a donation. There may be pressure from family members or even from themselves to donate. If there is any ambivalence on the donor's part, he or she may feel guilty. If the donor evaluation determines that the potential donor is not suitable, feelings of resentment from the recipient or his or her family may arise. Similar feelings may occur if, after donation, the recipient has an episode of rejection. It is important that potential donors, recipients, and their families be aware of these issues and have adequate support available if any occur. These supports come from the transplant team, mental health professionals, and close friends and family.

Of course, there are also many positive aspects to living donation. Although donating a part of the liver offers no direct medical benefit for the donor, it has significant advantages for the recipient. The surgery can be scheduled at a time when the recipient is in fairly good physical condition (timing is very important—the recipient should neither be too sick nor too well). Because LDLT is an elective operation, the surgery can be scheduled at a time that is convenient for both the donor and the recipient. A live donor transplant shortens the length of time the recipient must wait for an organ, usually shortens the hospital stay, and eliminates the stressful period of waiting for a suitable organ to become available.

Living donation also offers the donor and the recipient more time together, once the recipient becomes healthy again. This extra time enhances both parties' lives. The recipient can experience positive feelings, knowing that the gift came from a loved one. The donor can be comforted, knowing that he or she has helped not only a loved one but also another person on the waiting list, who can now receive a deceased donor organ that might have otherwise gone to the living donor recipient.

There is an extremely small risk of donor death due to the operation. This risk is estimated to be less than 0.2%, or 1 in 500. To date, three deaths have been reported in adult right lobe liver donors in the United States. Additionally, one live donor required transplantation soon after donation. There were no known similarities in the donors who died.

The average donor will be in the hospital for 7 to 10 days and will need to stay near the transplant program for approximately 1 week after discharge. The donor can recover at home but will need some assistance from friends and family as he or she recuperates from this major abdominal surgery. During the first few weeks after the surgery, the donor can accomplish many of the activities of normal living but will need help performing tasks that require lifting more than 5 pounds. Activity can be gradually increased over the next few weeks. The donor is typically out of work for 6 to 8 weeks depending on the type of work he or she does. For example, donors with sedentary jobs may be able to return to work at least part time in 6 to 8 weeks. Donors who perform manual labor usually need 8 to 12 weeks to recover.

Much like the recipient, the donor can expect some indirect expenses related to the evaluation and hospitalization. The donor's—or, more likely, the recipient's—health insurance will cover the donor's tests and physician and hospital expenses. Insurance companies rarely pay for the donor's transportation costs, food, lodging, child care expenses, or lost wages. Additional sources of funding, such as savings accounts, fundraisers, and the recipient, may be necessary to cover these costs. Coverage for postdonation complications varies from one insurance plan to the next and should be investigated before donation.

52. Are the results as good if I have a living donor compared with a cadaver donor?

Deceased donor liver transplantation has been the standard of care for patients with liver failure for more than 25 years. Hence, over time many transplant surgeons and programs have developed the skills and structure necessary to perform this operation successfully. This includes the ability to accept and list the most appropriate candidates, perform the surgery, assist in the recipient's recovery, and provide the necessary postoperative care and support. As a consequence, there is the expectation of excellent outcomes from cadaveric liver transplantation.

In the past 10 years adult living donor liver transplantation (LDLT) programs have been developed at hospitals with the goal of expanding the donor pool. Early reports showed that living donor recipients' outcomes were not as good as the outcomes experienced by their cadaver recipient counterparts. Later reports from LDLT programs with the most experience have now shown that LDLT can have at least equal, if not superior, outcomes. This increased effectiveness is likely attributable to the same factors that made deceased donor transplantation successful 20 years ago—experience in selecting appropriate recipients and donors, evolving surgical skill, and the infrastructure to optimize outcomes for all.

In addition, LDLT enjoys some other potential benefits over deceased donor transplantation. First, recipients may have an opportunity to undergo transplantation long before life-threatening liver-related events occur. They are likely to be in better physical and nutritional shape than patients awaiting cadaver donations. Second, the live donor liver, although smaller in size than a deceased donor liver, is more likely to have optimal donor characteristics due to the overall health of the donor. Third, the medical cost of the year before transplantation has been estimated to be approximately $100,000. By undergoing transplantation earlier in the course of the disease, much of this money can be saved. Finally, the use of live donor livers results in more deceased donor livers for patients in need of transplantation who do not have the option of LDLT. In some ways a living donor transplant may save two lives.

PART FIVE

Preparing for Transplantation

How do I need to prepare for transplantation?

I've heard that Tylenol is dangerous for the liver.
Is this true, and are there any medications
I need to avoid?

53. How do I need to prepare for transplantation?

If you have an active status on the transplant waiting list, it is important that your transplant team be able to contact you day and night, no matter where you are. There is a limited amount of time (60 minutes) during which the transplant team must decide whether to accept or decline an offer of a donor liver. If you cannot be contacted, the team will pass the liver on to the next candidate. Your transplant team may provide or suggest that you purchase a beeper. Make a list of people who need to be notified that you are having a liver transplant. Have someone make these calls while you are on the way to the hospital.

You may wish to consider packing an overnight bag in preparation for your hospitalization. You can include personal items, a bathrobe, slippers, and other items to make your stay more comfortable. You should leave valuables at home, however. You may need a phone card, credit card, or cell phone to make personal calls. Of course, you probably will not have to rush emergently to the hospital once you are called. Instead, you will likely have several hours to arrive—but packing a bag will be one less concern if you have already taken this step. If you are driving to the hospital, choose someone to drive you who will be available when the time comes. You may also wish to designate a back-up driver. Become familiar with the route to the hospital and where you need to go when you arrive. If you will be flying to the hospital, gather information on the flight schedules of several airlines and alternative travel options. You will also need a plan to get from the airport to the hospital.

If you have children, plan who will take care of them during your hospitalization. They may even need care plans that can begin in the middle of the night. If they are old enough to understand, talk to your children about your need for surgery and explain that you will be away from home during your hospitalization. Keep them abreast of the plans for their care while you are away.

It is important to establish a healthcare proxy, living will, or power of attorney before undergoing the transplantation procedure. Although the expectation with transplantation is rapid success, you may be incapacitated and unable to make decisions on your own behalf at some point. Discuss your wishes with your family or healthcare proxy so that these parties are fully informed and can carry out your plan. Your physician or social worker can help you with this difficult task.

Finally, take steps to ensure that you are in the best possible health before your surgery. Eat a healthy diet, take your medications, exercise, and talk about your feelings. Spend time with your family and friends, and avoid stress as much as possible.

While you are waiting for your transplant, you should try to remain as physically fit as possible. This will aid in your recovery. Even if you become weak and unable to leave your home, you can still exercise to some degree. Deep breathing, tightening and relaxing your muscles, stretching, and leg lifts are possible. You can try to do some light weightlifting with soup cans or rolls of coins. Walking is an excellent form of aerobic exercise that will help you maintain fitness and stamina.

It is important to be realistic about your goals. The longer you have been ill, the longer it will take you to regain your strength. This applies to both the patient awaiting transplantation and the recipient of a transplanted organ.

You may want to seek out the assistance of a physical therapist to set up a reasonable program with achievable goals. Your body will tell you when you are overdoing things. If you feel pain or excessive fatigue, you may have done too much and should rest. Even though the level of exercise may be light, it is important to warm up in the beginning and to cool down at the end. Stay well hydrated, albeit within the limits your doctor has recommended if you have fluid retention problems. You must realize that you will have "good" days and "bad" days, and you should adjust your workout accordingly.

You may wish to join a local health club or community center. Exercising with others can be motivational and keep you on a regular schedule. Try to schedule your exercise during your "best" time of day. For some people this is early in the day; for others exercising later is better. Also, try to vary your workouts to keep them interesting, because your level of fitness has a direct correlation with your recovery after transplantation.

In many diseases, adhering to a specific diet is helpful in controlling the progression of the disease. For example, patients with heart disease can reduce the risk of heart attack by following a low-fat, low-cholesterol diet. Unfortunately, no specific diets appear to benefit the liver directly. Instead, you should focus on eating a generally healthy diet with the recommended balance of food groups. Eating a healthy amount of fruits, vegetables, cereals, and meat provides you with the proper balance of carbohydrates, fats, and proteins. Some patients with liver disease have diminished appetites and require supplementation with small-volume, high-calorie, well-balanced liquid meals such as Ensure, Boost, and Sustacal. Eating more-frequent, smaller meals may be helpful as well.

Many patients with liver disease are prescribed dietary modifications to help them manage some of the side effects of cirrhosis. For example, patients with fluid retention (ascites or edema) may be on a low-sodium (approximately 2,000 milligrams per day) and fluid-restricted (approximately 2 liters or 67 ounces per day) diet. A dietitian from the liver transplant team can give you practical advice on how to meet these goals.

Patients with hepatic encephalopathy are often advised to significantly reduce their protein intake to gain better control of their encephalopathy. This recommendation can be dangerous and may result in severe protein malnutrition, which in turn may lead to muscle wasting, weakness, and poor wound healing. Although it is true that proteins are metabolized into more of the toxins responsible for hepatic encephalopathy compared with other food types, proteins are a necessary part of the diet. Patients with advanced liver disease are catabolic—that is, they are not adding fat and muscle to their bodies. Instead, the calories and energy brought in by their food intake are used to address the needs of the liver and other organs. In fact, these patients need *more* calories and proteins than healthy individuals just to maintain their weight and muscle mass. Thus any limitation of protein results in progressive loss of muscle and body weight.

Vitamin supplementation may also be necessary, particularly in patients with the cholestatic liver diseases of primary biliary cirrhosis and primary sclerosing cholangitis. These patients may become deficient in vitamins A, D, E, and K. If patients with liver disease can eat a healthy diet, then adding the standard multivitamins to the diet is usually not necessary.

54. I've heard that Tylenol is dangerous for the liver. Is this true, and are there any medications I need to avoid?

Almost all oral medications are absorbed into the bloodstream and carried immediately to the liver for processing. It is therefore important to avoid medications that can cause liver damage. Most prescription medications are safe for the liver, although some require a reduction in dose for patients with liver disease. If you have any questions about the safety of a new medication you have been prescribed, you should discuss your concerns with the prescribing physician and/or a member of the transplant team. Several commonly prescribed medications are worthy of specific mention in conjunction with liver disease.

Acetaminophen (Tylenol)

Acetaminophen is a medication that is available in both prescription strength and as an over-the-counter (OTC) drug. Acetaminophen is commonly combined with other pain medications such as oxycodone (Percocet), hydromorphone (Vicodin), and Darvocet. It is also found in many flu, cold, and headache preparations. Contrary to popular belief, acetaminophen can be taken safely by patients with liver disease, as long as they adhere to some limitations.

When swallowed, acetaminophen is absorbed into the blood and normally broken down into two parts: the part that controls flu and headache symptoms and a substance that is toxic to the liver. Fortunately, a detoxifier, called glutathione, is waiting for the toxin to arrive in the liver. Glutathione is rapidly, but not instantaneously, reproduced by the liver. The damaged liver may have a slower rate of glutathione production but nonetheless has a replenishable supply. Acetaminophen in doses up to 2,000 milligrams per 24 hours can be effectively detoxified even by the cirrhotic liver. It is important to note that acetaminophen does not slowly damage the liver and that it cannot cause cirrhosis. Because acetaminophen is found in many common medications, you should recognize that the total daily dose may come from different sources of acetaminophen.

Cholesterol-Lowering Agents

Cholesterol control has improved dramatically since the introduction of the cholesterol-lowering agents known as statins. One of the side effects of this class of drugs is liver cell toxicity, although this problem occurs in only a minority of patients. For patients with liver disease these drugs can be used with caution. First, however, you should determine whether a reduction in your cholesterol level is required. Lowering your cholesterol level reduces your risk of stroke and heart attack over the course of many years. For most patients with advanced liver disease this may not be a priority, so use of the statins can be avoided until after transplantation. Other patients may have a strong family history of coronary artery disease and stroke or may have had a heart attack themselves; in this group the statins may be necessary therapy. If a potentially liver-toxic drug is deemed to be of benefit to a particular patient, levels of the liver enzymes can be followed closely to confirm that liver toxicity is not occurring. These tests should be performed several times over the first 3 months of prescription use and then periodically thereafter. If the enzyme levels rise significantly above the baseline and remain high, the medication should be stopped.

Psychiatric Medications

Like the cholesterol-lowering agents, many psychiatric medications—but particularly the older ones—have the potential to cause liver damage. This effect occurs only rarely with use of the newer selective serotonin reuptake inhibitors such as Prozac, Paxil, and Celexa. Again, if a potentially liver-toxic drug is deemed to be of benefit to a particular patient, the liver enzyme levels can be followed closely to rule out liver toxicity. These tests should be performed several times over the first 3 months of prescription use and then periodically thereafter. If the enzyme levels rise significantly above the baseline and remain high, the medication should be stopped.

PART SIX

Surgery

How long will my liver transplant operation take?

55. *How long will my liver transplant operation take?*

Liver transplant surgery can take as little as 4 hours or as long as 12 to 15 hours. Many factors determine the length of the operation, including the experience of the surgical transplant team, the number of surgeries the recipient has undergone in the past, and the degree of the recipient's illness.

In the preoperative holding area, you will meet the anesthesiologist who will care for you during your operation and sign a consent form to permit him or her to give you anesthesia for the operation. A lot of activity will occur in this area as the medical staff prepares you for the surgery. Intravenous (in the vein) and arterial (in the artery) lines are placed in your arm and neck. These lines will still be in place when you wake up after the surgery. Electrocardiogram leads are placed on your chest to monitor your heart as well. All these preparations are needed to perform the transplant operation safely. When these preparations are complete, you will be wheeled into the operating room on a stretcher for your transplant operation.

Your operation will be appropriately timed for the arrival of your organ. The anesthesiologist will give you intravenous medication to put you to sleep. The anesthesia team will monitor your blood pressure, heart rate, breathing, and blood chemistries very closely during the entire operation.

After you are asleep, a breathing tube (endotracheal, or ET, tube) is placed in your throat and connected to a machine (ventilator) that breathes for you while you are asleep. A soft, small tube, called a Foley catheter, is inserted into your urinary bladder to drain your urine.

A soft tube may also be inserted through your nose or mouth that goes into your stomach; this nasogastric (NG) tube is used to keep your stomach empty to prevent vomiting and choking.

Your surgeon makes an incision that is either shaped like an upside-down "Y" or a hockey stick. The longer portion will be about 12 inches long, extending from the lower right side of the rib cage to just below the breast bone. The shorter portion will be 3 to 4 inches long, extending along the left lower rib cage (**Figure 9**).

Depending on your liver disease and your physical condition at the time of your transplant, your surgeon will use one of two methods to keep blood away from the liver area (to decrease bleeding) during the operation.

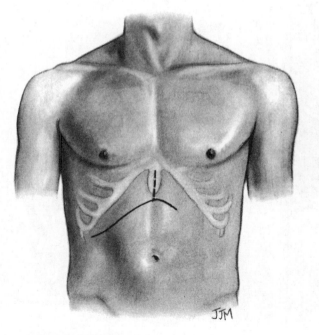

Figure 9   The upper abdomen.

Source: Illustration courtesy of Roger Jenkins, MD, who holds the rights.

In the piggyback technique, the blood vessels around the liver are clamped (held shut) while your new liver is sewn onto a part of your old blood vessel circulation. In a less frequently used procedure called venovenous bypass (**Figure 10**), a catheter (a small tube) is placed in a vein in your groin. Blood flows through this tube and through a machine that returns the blood to you through a catheter in a vein in your armpit. If the venovenous method is used, you will have two small punctures—in your armpit and in your groin—and a segment of your major blood vessels will be removed along with your old liver.

How your surgeon reconstructs your common bile duct depends on your liver disease. In most instances the ends of the original common bile duct and the donor

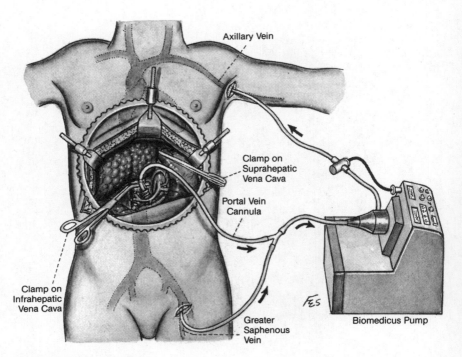

Figure 10   Venovenous Bypass.

Source: Illustration courtesy of Roger Jenkins, MD, who holds the rights.

common bile duct are sewn together (**Figure 11**). In this case a temporary tube or stent is placed in the common bile duct to permit doctors to x-ray the bile ducts after the surgery is complete. This tube is brought outside of your body through a small incision in your abdomen. The part of the tube that remains outside of your body connects to a bag into which the bile—a green/gold-colored fluid produced by your new liver—drains.

Finally, your surgeon will place three drains in your abdomen around your new liver, called Jackson-Pratt drains. One part is inside of your body, and the other is outside. The purpose of these drains is to draw excess fluids away from your liver. Your incision will be closed with staples and covered with a gauze dressing. The drains will be attached to your skin to hold them securely

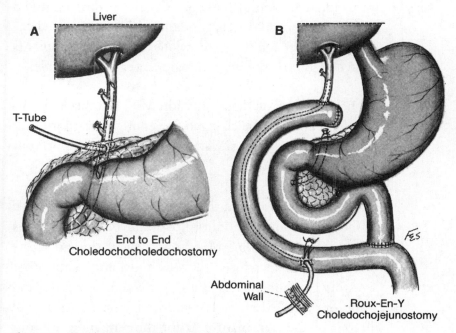

Figure 11   The bile duct after liver transplantation.

Source: Illustration courtesy of Roger Jenkins, MD, who holds the rights.

in place when you are moved. You will go directly to a postanesthesia care unit after the operation.

You will be given general anesthesia for the operation so you will have no recollection of the surgery or the time just before when you were in the preparation area. After the surgery is complete, you initially go to the postanesthesia care unit or to the intensive care unit (ICU) so that the doctors and nurses can monitor you very closely. When you wake up, you may hear unfamiliar sounds, such as the ventilator that may be helping you breathe and the machines that are monitoring your heartbeat, blood pressure, and breathing. You will not be able to talk if you have a breathing tube in place when you awaken. Some medications may make you very sensitive to the noises around you. You might feel nauseated from the anesthesia you were given to put you to sleep; you will be given medication for relief of this nausea. In addition, you may have some pain and discomfort from the surgery and will be given medication to help relieve it. Previous transplant recipients have described the incision pain as very manageable.

The dressing on your incision will be checked frequently and may be changed. It is not unusual for fluids to drain from your incision for some time after your operation.

Doctors and nurses in the postanesthesia care unit and ICU continuously monitor how well your new organ is functioning by taking blood tests, measuring and testing the fluids produced by your body, and using other testing methods, such as x-rays, when necessary and appropriate. When your condition is stable, you will move to the transplant unit for the remainder of your hospital stay.

Remember that many of the tubes, intravenous lines, and monitoring devices that were placed after you went to sleep will still be in place when you wake up. Any drains that were placed during the surgery will be in place as well.

Breathing Tube (Endotracheal Tube)

The tube that was placed in your throat and attached to the ventilator to help you breathe may still be in place when you wake up. While it is in place, fluid from your mouth and the tube will be removed frequently using a suction device. You will not be able to speak while the endotracheal (ET) tube is in place, but your nurse can help you communicate. You may want to establish a way to communicate with your loved ones, such as blinking your eyes once for "yes" and twice for "no." Trying to relax and letting the respirator do the work for you will conserve your energy and make having the tube in place more comfortable. Remember that the ET tube is temporary and necessary for your recovery.

The breathing tube is removed when the anesthesia has worn off completely and your physicians know that your lungs can function on their own. After a liver transplant the ET tube usually is removed within 8 to 24 hours after your surgery. Your doctors and nurses determine when you are ready to breathe on your own by performing a chest x-ray and taking blood samples to measure the oxygen in your blood. After the tube is removed, you may have a mild sore throat; the soreness disappears in a few days.

After the ET tube is removed, you will be encouraged to cough and breathe deeply very frequently to keep your lungs clear of fluids and to help oxygen flow freely.

Having someone support (splint) your stomach and back with a hand or a pillow helps make coughing less painful. Respiratory therapists and your nurses will assist you in keeping your lungs clear with chest therapy (gentle tapping of the lung area) and a spirometer (a device that helps you breathe deeply). All these precautions are intended to prevent fluid and secretions from collecting in your lungs and causing a lung infection or pneumonia.

Nasogastric Tube

If a nasogastric (NG) tube was inserted through your nose and into your stomach to keep your stomach empty, it still will be in place when you wake up. This tube is removed when your bowel sounds return or when you pass gas on your own, which usually happens within 24 to 72 hours of your operation.

Intravenous Lines

The intravenous (IV) lines may remain in place for most of your hospital stay. They enable your caregivers to draw your blood for tests, administer any medications that may be needed during your recovery, and provide fluids that help your blood circulate. They also are helpful in monitoring your heart and lung function.

Foley Catheter

The tube that was placed in your bladder to drain your urine will still be in place when you wake up. It generally is removed a few days after surgery.

Electrocardiogram Leads

When you leave the postanesthesia care unit or ICU, the electrocardiogram (ECG) leads that have been monitoring your heart are removed.

Jackson-Pratt Drains

The three Jackson-Pratt drains that your surgeon placed around your new liver will still be in place when you wake up. These tubes enter your abdomen through small incisions. Outside of the body, they look like clear plastic tubes with suction bulbs attached at the end. The fluid in the bulbs may be clear, yellow, or tinged with blood. All these colors are normal. Generally, two of these drains are removed within 24 hours of your surgery. The remaining Jackson-Pratt drain is removed within 10 days of your surgery.

Bile Tube

The tube that was placed in your bile ducts will still be in place when you wake up. It permits the doctors to monitor how well your new liver is working and how well the new bile ducts are healing. The bile tube is clamped shut when a blood test indicates that your bilirubin is less than 3 micromoles per liter (µmol/L) as measured in your blood. It will be removed during an office visit about 8 to 12 weeks after your surgery.

PART SEVEN

After Transplantation

What happens after I am discharged
from the hospital?

Can I drink alcohol after my transplant?

How long will my liver last after transplantation?

More . . .

56. What happens after I am discharged from the hospital?

Even before your surgery took place, the transplant team has made sure you are well prepared to be at home. If you have any questions or concerns, never hesitate to call a transplant team member—the doctor, nurse coordinator, or social worker. You have a lot of information to learn and understand.

After your transplant you may feel anxious, frightened, and overwhelmed. It will take some time for your energy level to return to normal and for you to settle into the routines you need to follow to stay well. Although other people may assume you are healthy now that the surgery is over, remember that you need to be patient during this recovery phase and follow the advice of your doctors and nurses. You will feel better as time goes on—but it takes time. You may have some setbacks along the way and feel discouraged. Share your feelings with your family, others who are close to you, and your doctors and nurses. If you are concerned about what you are feeling, you may want to consider seeing a mental health professional. If so, your doctors, nurses, or social worker can refer you to someone near your home.

Follow-up Visits

An appointment with a transplant surgeon or physician is scheduled before you leave the hospital. It is very important to keep this appointment and future appointments so that your progress can be checked, your medications reviewed, and your laboratory tests monitored to confirm that you and your new organ are doing well. You may need blood tests at a laboratory near your home and/or at the hospital between visits as well.

Other tests, such as x-rays or a biopsy, may need to be performed at certain times, too. Your visits are typically scheduled once a week for 1 to 2 months after transplantation. They are then spaced every 2 weeks, then once a month, then once every 6 to 8 weeks, and finally once every 3 to 6 months. You also may have appointments with your gastroenterologist or primary care physician.

Medicines

You will be taking several medicines after your transplant (described in detail in Section 4: Medications). When you leave the hospital, you will be given a medication card that lists which medicines you are taking, what doses to take, and when to take them. At your follow-up visits your doctor and transplant nurse coordinator review your medications and discuss any concerns you have, including side effects you might be experiencing. Because medications are sometimes adjusted to achieve the best results with the fewest side effects, it is important to bring your medication card to your follow-up appointments to record any changes.

Your responsibilities regarding your medications are summarized here:

- Make sure you take your antirejection medications, as well as your other medications, at the same time every day.
- If you missed or vomited a dose of your antirejection medicine and do not know what to do, call your transplant team.
- Do not use any over-the-counter medicines, except Tylenol (acetaminophen, but no more than 2,000 milligrams in 24 hours), without checking with your doctor or nurse.

- Do not use alcohol, cocaine, heroin, or marijuana—they may put your transplant at risk.
- Call the transplant team if you have any questions or concerns about your medicines.

Your Daily Record

It is wise to keep a daily record of your weight, temperature, frequency of urination and bowel movements, tube drainage, blood sugars (if you are diabetic), and any other notes. You should aim for accuracy when keeping this record, because it helps you identify signs of a problem and helps your doctors and nurses monitor your progress.

Your responsibilities regarding your daily record are summarized here:

- Fill in the information on your daily record sheet consistently and accurately. For example, take your temperature once a day at the same time of day.
- Weigh yourself at the same time every day on the same scale with the same amount of clothing on.
- Check the color and odor of your urine.
- Check your incision and tube site for an increase in redness and unusual drainage. Measure the amount of fluid draining from your tube site if you have one.
- Test your blood sugar at least two times a day: in the morning (this is called a fasting blood sugar) and in the late afternoon (only for those patients who have been advised to do so).
- Be sure to write down all of this information every day.

What to Watch for and When to Call the Transplant Team

While you were in the hospital, your doctors and nurses were constantly watching for signs of a rejection episode, infection, and other problems. Now that you are at home, you need to be a partner in your care and watch for these signs yourself. If you experience any of the following symptoms or if you "just don't feel right," call your transplant team:

- Temperature higher than 100.5°F
- Flu-like symptoms, such as chills, aches, joint pain, headache, and increased fatigue
- Nausea, vomiting, and diarrhea
- Severe stomach cramps
- Increased pain, redness, or tenderness over your transplant site
- Abnormal drainage near or on your incision
- Very dark or tea-colored urine
- Decrease in the amount of urine or no urine at all
- Pain or burning when urinating
- Frequent urination
- Light or clay-colored stools
- Yellowing of your eyes or skin
- A 6-pound weight gain in less than 3 days
- Abnormal blood sugars (if applicable)

Here are more reasons to call the transplant team:

- You cannot or did not take your antirejection medications.
- Your drainage tube comes out.
- You are short of breath or have chest pain.
- You have persistent stomach pain or indigestion.
- You catch a cold or another illness.
- Your urine is cloudy, bloody, or smells bad.
- You have been exposed to chickenpox, measles, German measles, or mumps and have never had the disease.
- You lose 3 pounds in less than 1 day.

- You have increased swelling in your hands or feet.
- Your doctor changes a medication or prescribes a new medication.
- You have sores or blisters in your mouth.
- You see white spots on your tongue or in your mouth.
- You want to take an over-the-counter medication other than acetaminophen (Tylenol).
- You have questions.

57. Can I drink alcohol after my transplant?

Virtually all liver transplant programs prohibit the use of alcohol after transplantation. Much of your own effort and the efforts of your family and physicians will be dedicated to keeping your liver healthy. This program includes proper nutrition, medications, and exercise. The deliberate ingestion of alcohol is in direct opposition to this goal. If your transplanted liver is destroyed by alcohol use, it is extremely unlikely that you would be accepted for a second liver transplant.

58. How long will my liver last after transplantation?

After undergoing liver transplantation, the expectation is that your liver will last for the rest of your life. It has been said that the liver does not age. That explains why it is perfectly acceptable to put a 70-year-old cadaveric donor liver into a 30-year-old recipient. This adage reflects a unique property of the liver: It is the only organ that is capable of regeneration. In other words, damaged liver cells are normally replaced by healthy functional cells. This process does not seem to decrease enough during a lifetime to result in a poorly functioning liver attributable only to the aging process.

Recurrence of liver disease (see Question 60) may limit the liver's ability to function indefinitely in the transplant recipient, however. Other life-limiting factors include conditions common to everyone—for example, heart disease, accidents, stroke, and cancer. To accurately address the question about survival after liver transplantation, several universally accepted milestones have been developed:

- *Operative mortality:* More than 90% of patients are still alive 30 days after liver transplantation. The reasons for operative mortality include anesthetic complications, excessive bleeding from varices during the operation, postoperative infections, hepatic artery thrombosis, and primary graft nonfunction.
- *One-year mortality:* More than 85% of patients are still alive 1 year after transplantation. The typical causes of death during this time frame are infections, delayed hepatic artery thrombosis, and bile duct problems resulting in jaundice and infection.
- *Three-year mortality:* Usually, 70% to 80% of patients are still alive 3 years after transplantation. Causes of death include recurrent disease, bile duct problems, chronic rejection, and, less likely, infections.
- *Five-year mortality:* Approximately 60% to 70% of patients are still alive 5 years after transplantation. Recurrent disease, chronic rejection, heart disease, and kidney failure are the major causes of death in this group.
- *Ten-year mortality:* Approximately 45% to 60% of patients are still alive 10 years after transplantation. Recurrent disease, chronic rejection, accidents, heart disease, stroke, kidney problems, and other cancers are the primary causes of death.

Note that after 10 years approximately 50% of liver transplant recipients are still alive. To have assessed this group for survival, by definition they must have been transplanted in the early 2000s. Since that time we have seen many advances in surgical techniques, postoperative care, ICU care, and immunosuppression. Additionally, transplant physicians have become more aware of long-term complications and, therefore, manage these problems more aggressively than in the past. It is expected that liver transplant recipients from the 2010s will have better long-term survival than their counterparts from the 1990s and 2000s.

You need time to regain your strength and endurance after your transplant, but eventually your activity level should get back to normal. It may take anywhere from 6 weeks to 6 months before you regain enough strength to return to work or to school. It might be possible to reduce your hours when you first return to work. Follow these guidelines when you get home:

- Do the muscle-toning exercises that you began in the hospital two times every day.
- Do not lift anything that weighs more than 10 to 15 pounds—including babies, children, and groceries—until you have been home from the hospital for 2 months. After 2 months you may gradually begin to lift heavier items if it does not cause discomfort around your incision.
- Walking and stair climbing are excellent exercises for maintaining muscle tone and strength. Consider walking 5 to 10 minutes a day when you first get home, slowly increasing the time you walk each week.
- Do not engage in any strenuous exercise, such as contact sports, jogging, tennis, or body conditioning (weightlifting, push-ups, sit-ups) for at least 2 months after you go home. Talk to your transplant doctor or nurse before you resume these types of activities.

- It is normal to tire easily. Pace yourself and rest when you are tired.
- Talk to your transplant team before you make any travel plans. They can help you maintain the routines you need to follow when you are away and instruct you on what to do if you need medical attention. They also can give you guidelines that will help you avoid infection and other problems when you are away from home.

You can resume sexual activity as soon as you feel able; there are no restrictions. Because you have been through a difficult surgery and are still recovering, it may take several months for your level of sexual desire to return to what you and your partner consider acceptable. Some medicines you are taking might also interfere with sexual functioning. Talk to your transplant team or primary care physician about any problems or concerns you may have. If you are sexually active and do not have a regular partner, you should practice safe sex by using condoms to reduce your risk of sexually transmitted diseases, such as chlamydia, syphilis, herpes, hepatitis, gonorrhea, and AIDS.

The following are things you can do (or avoid doing) to decrease your chance of an infection developing. Your transplant doctor or nurse will tell you when some of these restrictions may be lifted:

- Stay away from people who are obviously sick with the flu or a cold.
- Wash your hands with soap and water before you eat and after you go to the bathroom.
- Shower or bathe regularly. Wash your incision as you would any other part of your body. Do not use lotions or powders on your incision.

After Transplantation

- Clean cuts and scrapes with soap and water, and apply an antiseptic and a bandage to them.
- Do not, under any circumstances, change the litter in the cat box or bird cage without gloves. This could cause a serious infection.
- Do not garden, dig in dirt, or mow the lawn without gloves for 6 to 8 weeks after your transplant. This could cause a serious infection.
- Brush and floss your teeth daily.
- Keep your fingernails and toenails clean and trimmed. If your toenails are hard to manage or are ingrown, see a foot specialist.
- Talk to your doctor about getting the flu vaccine and the pneumonia vaccine. These do not contain a live virus and are safe for you to receive.
- Do not get any vaccine that contains a live virus, such as the smallpox or polio vaccine.
- Talk to your doctor if someone in your house received a live virus, such as the oral polio vaccine or diphtheria vaccine, if you have not already been vaccinated.
- Do not expose yourself to smoke—either first hand or second hand.
- Do not use alcohol.

59. Can I meet the family of my liver donor?

Recipients of donated organs often want to find out specifics about the person who donated the organ they received. In contrast, one of the basic tenets of organ donation is anonymity. This secrecy is necessary to protect the surviving family members' privacy. The donor family has likely experienced a traumatic event and the premature loss of a loved one. They may not be ready to meet a stranger who is living because of their loss. Sometimes, at a later date, many families who donate their relative's organs wish to know where and to whom the organs went.

Although there are no laws that prohibit donors and recipients from meeting, all OPOs have established privacy policies to protect both parties to the donation. However, this right to privacy may be waived if the two groups agree to meet.

The mechanism for meeting is initiated by writing a letter. The recipient is encouraged to write a letter to the donor family expressing his or her gratitude, hopes, and wishes for the future. The OPO, during its postdonation discussion with the donor family, makes them aware that the recipient may write letters to the donor family that will be kept at the OPO. Some families leave instructions with the OPO to not forward any such letters, because they do not want to reexperience the pain of losing their loved one. If the donor family wishes to know whether a letter is waiting for them, they can contact the OPO. The OPO can then forward the letter with all names removed. If the two parties interact frequently (always via the OPO), they may choose to meet. In these special circumstances where both parties want to meet and talk and both waive the right to privacy, a joint session is occasionally arranged by the OPO with the assistance of a specially trained chaperone.

A meeting between the donor family and the recipient can have long-lasting, powerful effects on both. Sometimes, bonds are made and communication is frequent. At other times the interaction is uncomfortable and terminated. Remember—every family grieves differently.

PART EIGHT

Complications

Can my original disease recur in the new liver?

What is acute rejection of the liver?

60. Can my original disease recur in the new liver?

Liver transplantation was performed because your liver disease caused cirrhosis and later signs of liver failure such as variceal bleeding, ascites, or encephalopathy. In most cases this process takes years to occur. Many liver diseases—particularly inherited diseases such as hemochromatosis, Wilson's disease, and alpha-1 antitrypsin deficiency—are cured by transplantation and therefore do not recur. Other diseases, such as alcoholic liver disease, do not recur as long as the recipient remains sober. Fatty liver disease, also known as nonalcoholic steatohepatitis, may not recur if the recipient maintains adequate weight and blood sugar control after transplantation.

Many of the common liver diseases are due to autoimmune processes. In other words, the immune system identifies the liver cells or bile ducts as foreign tissue and abnormal. It then tries to attack and eliminate the liver. This process results in slow but steady damage to liver and/or bile duct cells and can lead to cirrhosis. Examples of autoimmune liver diseases include autoimmune hepatitis, primary biliary cirrhosis, primary sclerosing cholangitis, and overlap syndrome. The pretransplant treatment of these conditions is difficult and may involve suppression of the immune system.

After transplantation, there is a risk—estimated to be 5% to 25%—that these autoimmune diseases may recur. Of course, there are also several reasons why the disease would *not* recur. After transplantation the patient takes immunosuppressive drugs, primarily to prevent rejection. Fortunately, these same drugs have a second benefit: They can be effective in controlling autoimmune diseases. A second reason for optimism regarding recurrence relates to the new liver's genetics. Before transplantation the recipient's immune system had recognized its own liver as foreign and developed specific antibodies to attack it. These antibodies may have been capable of recognizing only the native (recipient's own) liver; as a consequence, they may not identify the new liver as foreign. These antibodies are not the same ones that might potentially cause rejection of the transplanted organ.

There are other, equally valid, reasons why the autoimmune disease *might* recur in the new liver. First, the antibodies developed for the native liver may, in fact, be able to recognize the new liver as foreign, starting the disease process all over again. Second, the immune system may develop new antibodies to attack the transplanted liver. Third, the transplant team and patient are usually motivated to reduce the immunosuppressive medications in an effort to limit the side effects; as a result, the autoimmune disease may become inadequately controlled by the medications. Finally, there may be other factors that we are not aware of that cause autoimmune diseases.

Recurrence of hepatitis C virus (HCV) disease in the transplanted organ occurs in all patients transplanted for HCV-related cirrhosis who still have the virus when they undergo transplantation. This virus is actually detectable in the bloodstream and the new liver as early as during the transplant operation. Typically, HCV-infected patients develop elevated liver enzymes and signs of an inflamed liver about 3 to 6 months after the transplant. Most of these patients have mild to moderate inflammation, minimal to mild scarring of the liver, and acceptable 1- and 5-year survival rates. Most can expect 10 to 20 years of good liver health before significant damage from

HCV recurs. A smaller proportion of patients, perhaps 20% to 40%, develop a more rapid progression of HCV liver disease. These patients may develop signs of liver failure 5 to 10 years after the transplant. Even less common (affecting 1% to 5% of HCV-infected patients) is fibrosing cholestatic hepatitis, which can destroy the new liver within 1 year. At the present time we have not identified any pretransplant features that can predict with certainty which pathway any individual liver transplant recipient with HCV disease will follow.

Patients transplanted with known HCV are monitored in the usual posttransplant fashion. Some transplant programs schedule liver biopsies to occur at predetermined time intervals to get an idea of the rate at which inflammation and scarring are progressing. Other programs biopsy only those patients who develop abnormal liver blood tests. If the biopsy shows significant inflammation or scarring due to recurrent HCV, treatment is considered.

There are three approaches to treating hepatitis C recurrence after liver transplantation:

- Prophylaxis against hepatitis C is the administration of medications to protect the new liver from becoming infected with the virus. Unfortunately, no HCV antibody preparations effectively protect the new liver, so this approach is not possible.
- The preemptive approach calls for treatment of everyone with hepatitis C after transplantation, regardless of the timing or severity of the infection.
- Treatment of established recurrent disease is the most commonly applied option.

To date, no published study has compared preemptive therapy to treatment of established disease. In addition, no data suggest that early treatment during the first clinical signs of recurrent HCV disease influences the natural history of the disease. Based on the limited available data, the role for preemptive antiviral therapy remains to be defined.

A number of recent studies have reported that combination therapy with interferon and ribavirin is associated with a sustained virologic response (cure) rate of 20% to 30% in liver recipients with recurrent HCV disease; however, most of these studies were small. One major problem with these studies is the significant variability in the ways that patients were chosen for treatment and immunosuppression, making the interpretation of the results of these studies difficult. Nevertheless, the rate of sustained virologic response seems to be lower than the rate reported for nontransplant HCV patients. In addition, interferon/ribavirin therapy in liver recipients with recurrent HCV disease is associated with toxicity of the medications and side effects, leading to more frequent dose reductions and discontinuation of therapy.

In view of the many unknowns about the natural history of recurrent HCV disease, two approaches to treatment can be suggested. The first approach is to start treatment at the first evidence of acute graft injury (acute recurrent HCV disease), which typically occurs in the first 6 months after transplant. The second approach is to initiate treatment when the patient shows evidence of liver disease based on the results of a liver biopsy. Given that the results of treatment at these two time points, the tolerability of the treatment, and its effectiveness in improving the transplant recipient's health are unknown, it is important to discuss these issues with your transplant team. Your transplant team may already have a preferred approach.

Many questions remain unanswered with regard to the treatment of post–liver transplant HCV disease, including the timing of treatment, the best treatment regimen, the most effective duration of therapy, and the role of immunosuppression in progressive recurrent HCV disease. Nevertheless, although no firm recommendations can be made, the research conducted to date suggests that a patient with recurrent HCV disease who has stage 2 or higher fibrosis should be considered for a trial of combination pegylated interferon/ribavirin therapy. Several ongoing studies are currently addressing these issues.

61. What is acute rejection of the liver?

Rejection is a signal that your immune system has identified your new liver as foreign tissue and is trying to get rid of it. Preventing rejection with immunosuppressive medications is the first priority. An episode of rejection of the transplanted liver is very common, occurring in as many as 60% of liver recipients. Most people experience a rejection episode within 5 to 10 days of the transplant operation. The signs you and your doctors and nurses are watching for include a low-grade temperature, decreased appetite, abdominal discomfort, joint and/or back pain, tenderness over the liver, increased abdominal fluid, and feeling like you might have the flu. Other signs include an elevation of your liver function blood tests, a change in the color of your bile (from dark green to light yellow), and a decrease in the amount of bile produced.

Because most people do not have obvious signs of rejection, your liver function tests are monitored closely. If they are abnormal, a liver biopsy may be performed to confirm that you are experiencing a rejection episode. A liver biopsy is accomplished at the hospital bedside.

The upper part of your incision is closed by staples, which are removed several days after your surgery. This permits access to the new liver by a biopsy needle. A liver biopsy usually is not painful, but you will feel pressure when the needle is inserted into the liver. Liver biopsies also can be performed on an outpatient basis. This kind of procedure may be necessary if your liver function tests rise after you go home from the hospital.

If you have an episode of rejection, the amount of anti-rejection medication you are taking will be increased or a different combination of antirejection medications will be prescribed. In almost all cases, *adjusting the medications will stop the rejection episode.*

Heart Transplantation

PART ONE

The Basics

What are the causes of heart failure?

How is heart failure treated?

What is a ventricular assist device (VAD)?
When should patients with heart failure be
considered for a VAD?

More . . .

62. What is heart failure?

The heart is a powerful muscle, approximately the size of your fist, that pumps blood throughout the body. The left side of the heart receives blood from the lungs that is full of oxygen and then pumps it out to the body, including all your organs, brain, limbs, and other body parts. After the body uses up the oxygen in the blood, the blood is returned back to the right side of the heart, where it is pumped to the lungs to receive more oxygen. The cycle then repeats itself.

Your heart consists of four chambers that hold the blood as it moves through the heart. The upper chambers are called atria. The lower chambers are called ventricles, and they do the main work of the heart, pumping blood out of the heart. There are four valves in the heart that act like one-way doors, separating the blood as it moves forward. Healthy valves open to let blood through and then close to keep blood from moving backward (**Figure 12**).

Heart failure

A chronic condition in which your heart cannot supply enough blood and oxygen to your body to keep up with your body's demands. Sometimes called "congestive heart failure" because it is often associated with fluid buildup, swelling, and difficulty breathing.

Heart failure means that your heart cannot supply enough blood and oxygen to your body to keep up with your body's demands. Sometimes heart failure is called "congestive heart failure" because it is often associated with fluid buildup, swelling, and difficulty breathing.

Heart failure is not a heart attack, which is when a sudden blockage occurs in one of the arteries that feeds the heart (known as the coronary arteries). This is usually associated with significant chest pain and can be a life-threatening emergency. In contrast, heart failure is often a chronic condition that can be present for a very long time. Patients with heart failure typically experience fluctuations and variations in the severity of their symptoms over time.

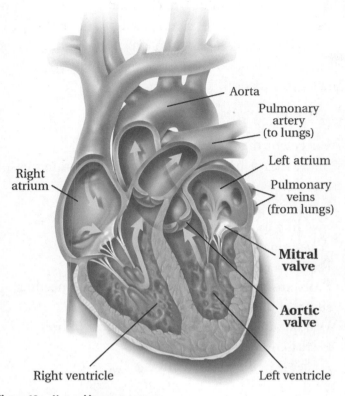

Right atrium

Aorta

Pulmonary artery (to lungs)

Left atrium

Pulmonary veins (from lungs)

Mitral valve

Aortic valve

Right ventricle

Left ventricle

Figure 12   Normal heart structures.

Source: Reprinted with permission from Lahey Clinic Foundation.

Heart failure is often classified into two categories: systolic dysfunction and diastolic dysfunction. Systolic dysfunction is when the heart muscle becomes enlarged and weakened. The weakened heart muscle doesn't pump enough blood forward when the ventricles contract. Diastolic dysfunction is when the heart muscle is not weakened but rather has become stiff. The stiff muscle can't relax between contractions, which prevents the heart chambers (known as ventricles) from adequately filling with enough blood. In either case the heart is not working efficiently.

The term "heart failure" refers to the various symptoms that patients may experience but does not explain the cause of their heart problem. Most patients who have heart failure do have some type of abnormality of their heart function.

The symptoms of heart failure are

- Fatigue or tiredness with little effort
- Shortness of breath with exertion, becoming easily breathless
- Loss of appetite or nausea
- Swelling in ankles or legs
- Abdominal bloating or fullness
- Rapid weight gain
- Problems breathing when lying flat, or needing to sit up or use extra pillows to sleep
- Waking up at night coughing or short of breath
- Increased nighttime urination
- A racing or skipping heartbeat

63. What is a cardiomyopathy?

The term cardiomyopathy literally means "abnormal heart muscle." This refers to the abnormal function of the heart itself and does not refer to the effect on the body or any symptoms.

Most patients who have symptoms of heart failure indeed have some type of cardiomyopathy. Their heart muscle has weakened and the heart has become dilated. The weakened heart muscle cannot pump blood efficiently and becomes tired easily.

In patients who have a cardiomyopathy, their weakened heart is pumping less blood with each contraction, so fluid backs up into the lungs. Also, less blood is pumped to the kidneys. The kidneys are the organs that regulate electrolytes and fluids in the body and help the body get rid of extra fluid. As a result, the body will have a tendency to become congested with fluid, which is why this condition may lead to symptoms known as "congestive heart failure."

There are several different causes of a cardiomyopathy. The most common cause is coronary artery disease (blocked arteries of the heart). This is known as an ischemic cardiomyopathy. All other cardiomyopathies are referred to as nonischemic. A nonischemic cardiomyopathy can be due to infections or viruses, alcohol abuse, high blood pressure, heart valve problems, or the toxic effects of certain drugs (such as certain cancer medications). A cardiomyopathy can also be inherited or may be due to congenital heart problems that were present at birth. Some patients may have developed an "idiopathic" cardiomyopathy, which means that the cause is unknown.

64. What are the causes of heart failure?

In most cases heart failure is caused by another health problem. Some of these problems damage the heart muscle, so the heart isn't able to pump as well as it should. Other problems make the heart work harder, which can weaken the heart by tiring it out.

Coronary artery disease (CAD) is the most common cause of heart failure. The coronary arteries are the small blood vessels that supply blood and oxygen to the heart muscle. CAD is caused by atherosclerosis (also called "hardening of the arteries"). This condition occurs when plaque (deposits of fat or cholesterol) accumulates on the inner surface of the arteries. As plaque builds up the coronary arteries may become

Coronary artery disease (CAD)

The most common cause of heart failure caused by atherosclerosis (also called "hardening of the arteries"). This condition occurs when plaque (deposits of fat or cholesterol) accumulates on the inner surface of the arteries, narrowing the coronary arteries and reducing blood flow to the heart muscle. As a result, the heart muscle, deprived of oxygen-rich blood, cannot work normally and can weaken, and heart failure may develop.

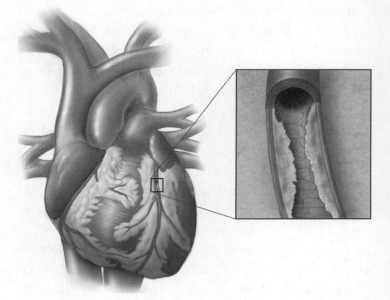

Figure 13   Coronary artery disease (CAD).

Source: Reprinted with permission from Lahey Clinic Foundation.

narrowed, and this reduces blood flow to the heart muscle (**Figure 13**). As a result the heart muscle that is deprived of oxygen-rich blood cannot work normally. The muscle can weaken, and heart failure may develop.

A heart attack can occur when the narrowing in a coronary artery progresses to the point where a part of or the entire artery is blocked. This is known as a myocardial infarction. This blockage can stop blood flow to a part of the heart muscle. Without the oxygen-rich blood, this part of the heart muscle may become permanently damaged. The damaged portion of the heart muscle loses its ability to pump, and scar tissue may develop. Therefore after a heart attack, the rest of the heart muscle must work harder. Over time, the strained heart muscle may weaken further, and heart failure can develop.

Blood pressure is a measure of how hard blood pushes against the artery walls. A normal blood pressure should be less than 130/80 mm Hg. High blood pressure (also called hypertension) is when blood is pushing harder than normal. This makes your heart work harder. As a result, over time the chambers of your heart may enlarge or may become abnormally thickened. Ultimately, if the high blood pressure is not controlled, the heart muscle becomes less efficient, and may stretch and weaken. This may lead to heart failure.

Valve disease occurs when the valves between the heart chambers do not open or close properly. If a heart valve becomes narrowed (known as "valve stenosis"), it does not open fully, and your heart has to work harder to pump the blood forward to your body. If a valve does not close tightly, blood leaks backward (referred to as "valve regurgitation"), forcing your heart to pump some of the same blood back through the same valve again. This backflow creates extra work for the heart and can weaken it. Over time, this can possibly lead to heart failure symptoms.

A **cardiomyopathy** is a weakening of the heart muscle. This is described in detail in Question 63. The dilated, weakened heart muscle cannot pump efficiently, and this can cause heart failure to occur.

Other health problems can strain the heart and make it more likely to weaken. Diabetes makes coronary artery disease and heart failure more likely. Heart failure may occur more commonly if you have abnormal thyroid function or a low blood count ("anemia"). Chronic kidney problems can affect how well your body handles its electrolytes and can lead to water retention, which may worsen symptoms of heart failure.

Cardiomyopathy

A weakening of the heart muscle due to inflammation ("myocarditis"), infections or viruses, alcohol abuse, the toxic effects of certain drugs, inherited or congenital heart problems, and "idiopathic" (unknown) causes.

65. What is the ejection fraction (EF)? If I have a low ejection fraction, does that mean that I need a heart transplant?

Ejection fraction (EF)

A measure of how well the heart pumps blood out of its chambers (ventricles).

The **ejection fraction (EF)** is a measure of how well the heart pumps blood out of its chambers (ventricles). With each contraction of your heart, a certain amount ("fraction") is pumped out of the heart ("ejected"). A normal ejection fraction is approximately 50% to 60%. In other words, a healthy heart ejects at least half of the blood from the ventricles with each beat.

Your ejection fraction can be measured by a number of different heart tests that look at your heart. Some examples include an echocardiogram (ultrasound of your heart), heart catheterization (invasive x-ray test of your heart using thin tubes), and certain types of stress testing that may include pictures of your heart (nuclear medicine x-ray pictures).

A patient who has a cardiomyopathy usually has a reduced ejection fraction. Fortunately, most patients who have a cardiomyopathy will not need to undergo heart transplantation. Interestingly, there are some patients who have a cardiomyopathy who have minimal or no symptoms at all.

Therefore most patients who have a low ejection fraction never need a new heart. Modern treatments now allow most patients to control their symptoms and live a full and healthy lifestyle. However, if a patient develops severe heart failure and becomes very sick, he or she may then need to be evaluated for heart transplantation.

66. How is heart failure treated?

Your treatment plan depends on your specific medical history. The goal of treatment is to relieve some of your symptoms and to help reduce the work your heart has to perform with each heartbeat. This helps to make your heart pump more efficiently.

The focus of your treatment includes lifestyle and dietary changes, exercise, important medications, and, sometimes, special implanted devices to help the heart. It is also important to treat any other associated medical condition that may be affecting your heart. This may include fixing blocked coronary arteries, repairing damaged heart valves, or correcting abnormal heart rhythms.

Your doctor will instruct you to carefully restrict the salt (sodium chloride) in your diet. A high-salt diet can increase your blood pressure but, more importantly, can cause your body to retain water. This can cause swelling and worsened symptoms. Changing what you eat and drink can help prevent fluid from backing up in your body.

Monitoring your health and weighing yourself daily is also an excellent way to stay healthy. Any rapid weight gain can be a sign that you are retaining water and may mean that your treatment plan may need to be adjusted. You should weigh yourself at the same time every morning with the same scale. Write your weight down each day, and call your doctor if you gain more than 3 pounds in one day or if you gain more than 5 pounds in a week. The dosage of your medications may need to be adjusted.

Your heart failure symptoms will improve if you stay as physically active as possible. Aerobic activities, such as walking, can help by exercising the heart and may allow it to get stronger. When you stay active, you may feel less tired and have fewer symptoms. It is a good idea to have a regular exercise schedule. By exercising regularly and keeping your body conditioned, you will feel better and can exercise longer.

Although it is important to stay active, your body also needs rest. Regular periods of both rest and exercise should be scheduled into your day. If you listen to your body, you will know when it needs rest or activity.

Medications are an essential component of your heart failure treatment. Certain medications can help you live longer by improving the way your heart pumps over time. Other medications can relieve symptoms and improve your quality of life (**Table 5**). It may be necessary to make frequent adjustments to these medications to find the combination of medications that works best for your condition.

Additionally, your heart failure may require the implantation of special devices, such as an implanted cardioverter defibrillator (ICD) or a biventricular pacemaker. In very rare cases a patient who has severe heart failure may need to have a special heart pump implanted, known as a ventricular assist device (VAD). These devices are addressed in the following sections.

67. What is an implanted cardioverter defibrillator (ICD)?

An **implanted cardioverter defibrillator (ICD)** is a small electronic device implanted permanently inside your body. It is like a pacemaker but has several extra features. It is usually inserted under the skin in the area of your upper chest, near your left shoulder (**Figure 14**). This procedure is performed by a cardiac electrophysiologist,

Implanted cardioverter defibrillator (ICD)

A small electronic device implanted permanently inside your body to continually monitor your heart rhythm (the pattern and speed of your heartbeat).

Table 5   Medications Used to Treat Heart Failure

Type of Medication	What It Does
ACE Inhibitor	• Reduces the strain on the heart and lowers blood pressure, making it easier for heart to pump. • Favorably alters hormones that can chronically damage the heart.
Beta-Blocker	• Slows the heart rate (pulse) and lowers blood pressure. • Favorably alters hormones that can chronically damage the heart. • May strengthen the pumping action of the heart.
Angiotensin Receptor Blocker (ARB)	• Reduces the strain on the heart and lowers blood pressure, making it easier for heart to pump. • Favorably alters hormones that can chronically damage the heart. • May be prescribed instead of an ACE Inhibitor.
Diuretic	• Also known as "water pills." • Helps the body get rid of extra water. This may improve breathing and reduce swelling.
Digoxin	• Can slow the heart rate and help the heart pump more blood with each contraction/heartbeat.
Aldosterone Antagonist	• Favorably alters hormones that can chronically damage the heart, which decreases the strain on the heart. • Used in cases of more severe heart failure.
Hydralazine and Nitrates	• Reduces how hard the heart has to work, and can lower blood pressure. • Two separate medications, used in combination. • May be prescribed instead of an ACE Inhibitor or ARB, if you are unable to tolerate them due to weakened kidney function.

who is a heart doctor that specializes in the electrical disturbances of the heart.

An ICD continually monitors your heart rhythm (the pattern and speed of your heartbeat). If your heart rhythm becomes too slow or too fast, the ICD sends out electrical signals to restore your rhythm back to normal. Depending on the type of abnormal heart rhythm, this electrical impulse is referred to as a "cardioversion" or a

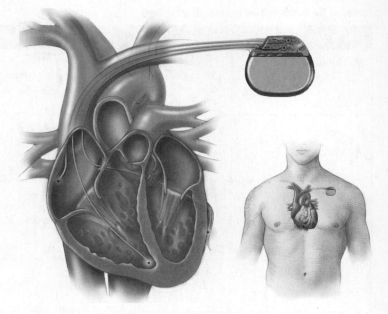

Figure 14   Implanted cardioverter defibrillator (ICD).

Source: Reprinted with permission from Lahey Clinic Foundation.

"defibrillation." Sometimes, these abnormal rhythms are very dangerous, and an ICD could save your life.

If your heartbeat becomes too slow (known as "bradycardia"), the ICD sends out electrical impulses to bring the rhythm back up to a normal rate. This is referred to as "pacing" and is the same feature that is found in a standard pacemaker. If your heartbeat becomes dangerously fast (known as "tachycardia"), the ICD can send impulses to slow it down. It can also deliver a small shock to return the heart back to a normal rhythm again.

If you have a cardiomyopathy or heart failure, you may be at increased risk of these dangerous arrhythmias (heart rhythm problems). Your doctor may recommend that you have an ICD implanted to protect you from any of these rare but serious life-threatening heart rhythm disturbances. If these dangerous abnormal heart rhythms are not corrected quickly, they could lead to cardiac arrest. An ICD can protect you from these problems.

68. What is a biventricular pacemaker (bi-V pacemaker)?

When you have heart failure, your heart is weakened and doesn't pump as well as it should. A cardiac resynchronization therapy (CRT) device may help your heart work better. CRT is also called "biventricular pacing." For many heart failure patients, a CRT device can reduce symptoms and improve their quality of life. Most biventricular pacemaker CRT devices also incorporate the extra technology and features of an implanted cardioverter defibrillator (ICD) as well. This is called a "biventricular ICD" or "CRT-ICD."

Your heart has an electrical system that controls its pumping action (called the "conduction system"). This system sends automatic electrical impulses through the heart muscle that tell the heart to beat properly. If you have heart failure, the heart muscle may be damaged, and these electrical signals may travel more slowly through this damaged muscle. This is referred to as a "conduction system delay," which is also known as a "bundle branch block." This abnormality can easily be detected on an electrocardiogram (ECG), which is a simple recording of your heart rhythm. About one-third of patients with a cardiomyopathy have a bundle branch block.

If you have a bundle branch block on your ECG, this may mean that the heart's pumping chambers (ventricles) may not be synchronized properly and may not be contracting together. If this happens, the heart

The Basics

becomes less efficient and less blood is pumped out to the body, which can make heart failure worse.

If your left and right ventricles are not contracting together and you have heart failure, a CRT device ensures that the contractions are timed correctly. Then, the two pumping chambers become resynchronized, and blood is pumped out of the heart more efficiently. Whereas a standard pacemaker or ICD contains only one or two wires ("leads") on the right side of the heart, a CRT device uses a third wire. This extra wire sends signals to the left side of the heart, so that the electrical impulses can stimulate both right and left ventricles simultaneously, thereby increasing the pumping force of the heartbeat.

Like an ICD, a CRT device is implanted by a cardiac electrophysiologist, who is a heart doctor that specializes in the electrical disturbances of the heart.

69. What is a ventricular assist device (VAD)? When should patients with heart failure be considered for a VAD?

Ventricular assist device (VAD)

A mechanical pump device that is surgically implanted to help maintain the pumping ability of a heart that has become so severely weakened it is unable to effectively function on its own.

A **ventricular assist device (VAD)** is a mechanical pump device that is surgically implanted to help maintain the pumping ability of a heart that has become so severely weakened that it is unable to effectively function on its own. In patients who have very severe heart failure and are eligible, these mechanical heart pumps can significantly improve their symptoms and their survival rate.

Most VADs that are implanted support the left side of the heart (left ventricle), because this is the main pumping chamber of the heart. These pumps are referred to as left ventricular assist devices (LVAD). There are also other pumps, used less frequently, that help both the left and right ventricles pump blood, known as biventricular assist devices (Bi-VAD).

The typical LVAD involves a tube that is surgically connected to the left ventricle and directs the blood from the ventricle into the pump (**Figure 15**). The pump then sends blood out into the aorta (the large blood vessel leaving the left ventricle, delivering blood to the entire body). This effectively bypasses the weakened ventricle but delivers a full amount of blood and oxygen to the body and all the vital organs.

The VAD is connected to a "system controller," which is connected to the tube that exits from the abdomen (the "driveline"). This is powered by an external battery pack.

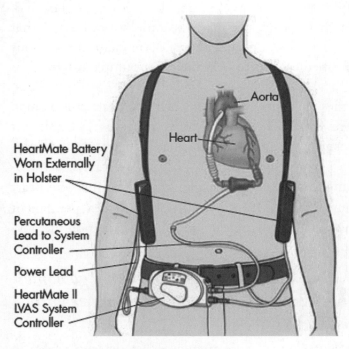

Figure 15 **Left ventricular assist device (LVAD).**

Source: Reprinted with permission from Thoratec Corporation.

A VAD must always be connected to its power source, either the portable battery pack or to the power base console, which is plugged into an electric wall socket.

The battery pack can be worn in a small holster, making it easy to move around without being "plugged" into the wall. Technologic advances in the portable battery pack have improved the quality of life and independence of patients who are now free to move around for several hours at a time with the portable pack. Many patients who are home with a VAD are capable of living an active lifestyle and to resume some of their normal routines and activities.

A heart failure patient can be considered for a VAD after all medical and device therapy has failed and the patient has developed severe end-stage heart failure. Often, these patients are unable to leave the hospital, and their heart may have become so weakened that they are now dependent on permanent intravenous (IV) medications to help the heart pump stronger.

In these patients a VAD may help the heart pump blood more effectively until a heart becomes available for transplantation (referred to as a "bridge to transplantation"). For others who do not qualify for heart transplantation but who are still suffering from severe heart failure, an LVAD may be implanted as a permanent pump to assist their heart, so-called destination therapy.

70. Can a patient with a VAD ever go home? What are the complications associated with use of a VAD?

Implantation of a ventricular assist device (VAD) in many patients results in a dramatic improvement in their medical condition and health. Heart failure symptoms can improve significantly. This allows most patients to return back home with the VAD, to enjoy an improved quality of life.

After surgery to implant the VAD, you will be monitored in the intensive care unit. Typically, a breathing tube will help your lungs function and can be removed within a few days. Within a week or so you will be moved out of the ICU to a regular hospital room.

After this surgery you will experience some pain where the incisions were made in your chest and abdomen. The medical staff will give you pain medicine in addition to your heart medicines. As you recover, you will work with nurses and physical therapists to regain your strength and mobility.

After this, you will learn how the VAD works. You will need to become intimately familiar with all the components of the VAD system. You will become comfortable performing all "troubleshooting" maneuvers.

Most patients are able to leave the hospital within 2 to 4 weeks of surgery, assuming their recovery is uneventful. Depending on the nature of your job, it may be possible to return back to work within several months after your VAD surgery.

Because the implantation of a ventricular assist device involves major heart surgery, there are important potential complications. There is a small risk of serious complications related to the VAD surgery itself, such as a heart attack, stroke, kidney failure, or even death. There is also a small chance that the VAD may not work properly, may malfunction, or may not improve your heart failure symptoms. In these situations a repeat VAD surgery may be necessary.

After successful VAD implantation, however, most patients do very well. Because there is a mechanical pump in the bloodstream, there is always a small risk of blood clots forming or a stroke developing; you will be maintained on some type of blood thinner to prevent this.

The greatest risk to a patient with a VAD is the risk of infection. This is usually a local skin infection where the tube (the "driveline") exits from your abdomen. Some patients, however, may develop a systemic infection ("sepsis") that can be very serious. Any type of infection is taken very seriously, as infection can lead to malfunction of the VAD, and this can jeopardize your health. You will learn techniques to meticulously care for your VAD and its components to minimize the risk of infection.

PART TWO

Before Transplantation

Who is a good candidate for heart transplantation?
Is there an age limit?

What are the indications for a heart transplant?
Why do I need a heart transplant?

What tests will I need to have before
I am considered for heart transplantation?

More...

71. Who is a good candidate for heart transplantation? Is there an age limit?

Before you have a heart transplant, a team of health care professionals will determine if you are healthy enough to receive a new heart. It is necessary to establish that you are sick enough to require a transplant but also to ensure that you are physically capable of having a transplant.

Most patients who are being considered for transplantation are less than 70 years of age before being listed for a heart transplant. Although patients up to the age of 70 may be considered for transplantation, those over the age of 65 years need to be in excellent physical condition in order to be considered. Over 50% of patients on the waiting list are over the age of 50, and 10% are over the age of 65.

To be considered for a heart transplant, the following basic questions about your heart failure condition need to be addressed:

- Have all other therapies been tried or excluded (including medications, corrective cardiac surgery, heart catheterizations, devices, etc.)?
- Are you likely to die without the transplant?
- Are you in generally good health other than the heart disease?
- Are there any active infections or cancer at the time of transplant?
- Are you severely obese? (Your weight must be proportionate to your height.)
- Do you have any evidence of significant vascular disease (narrowing in the arteries that supply the brain or legs)?

- Do you have any psychological problems that may interfere with your ability to take medications or to attend frequent follow-up doctor visits?
- Can you adhere to the lifestyle changes, including complex drug treatments and frequent examinations/procedures required after a transplant? (You will be a "patient" for the rest of your life.)
- Do you have some type of social or family network that can support you during your illness and your waiting period and during your recovery process after a potential transplant?
- Do you have some type of appropriate medical insurance?
- Are you free of alcohol, drug, and tobacco use?

If you answered "no" to any of the above questions, you may not be a suitable candidate for a heart transplant. Of course, each patient is considered individually, so that every patient is given full consideration.

72. What are the indications for a heart transplant? Why do I need a heart transplant?

Patients who are suffering from advanced (end-stage) heart failure but are otherwise healthy may be considered for a transplant. When a patient's heart disease and heart failure becomes advanced and very severe, sometimes it can no longer be improved by medications, implanted devices, or corrective cardiac surgery (valve surgery or bypass of the coronary arteries).

Generally speaking, a patient is referred for a cardiac transplant evaluation once his or her heart failure has progressed and has become so severe that the patient's prognosis has become very poor. When your condition becomes refractory to all standard therapy, heart transplantation can offer you the potential of living an independent and normal, active life once again. If you are eligible, a heart transplant can drastically improve your functional capacity, quality of life, and long-term survival.

Because of advances in surgical techniques and the improved medical management of transplant recipients, an increasing number of people can now have a heart transplant. Currently, the choice is mainly limited by the availability of a donor heart that is suitable for transplantation. Your candidacy is determined on an individual basis and involves many different factors.

After all your tests have been completed, your pre-transplant cardiologist presents your case to a heart transplant selection committee. This is a team that meets weekly and is composed of heart surgeons, cardiologists, transplant nurses, infection experts, and a social worker.

Your case is reviewed, and the committee discusses recommendations for the best course of treatment for you. In some cases you may be "too well" for listing at this time and may continue on medications. Other times a patient may need to be listed for transplant immediately. In other cases a patient may be determined not to be a candidate who will benefit from a heart transplant, because of one of several possible reasons.

73. What tests will I need to have before I am considered for heart transplantation?

A heart transplant is extraordinarily demanding on many levels. Because there are so many more candidates for transplants than there are available hearts, the transplant list must be carefully screened. A multidisciplinary team of heart doctors, surgeons, nurses, social workers, and bioethicists evaluates your medical history, diagnostic test results, social history, and psychosocial assessment. This is referred to as a formal pretransplant evaluation.

Extensive pretransplant testing is performed to assess whether any other treatment options exist for you, to determine if you are sick enough to require a transplant, and to ensure that you are physically capable of having a transplant. A careful search is conducted for any potential contraindications to a heart transplant, such as undiagnosed cancer or other serious medical problem. A description of many of the tests that are necessary follows:

- Blood tests
  - A series of blood tests are used to evaluate your liver function, kidney function, blood and tissue type, and any previous exposure to various infections. You will be tested for HIV, regardless of your risk factors.
- BNP laboratory test
  - This is a heart failure blood test. It measures the level of a hormone in your blood called B-type natriuretic peptide (BNP). Your heart's pumping chambers (ventricles) produce extra BNP when they can't pump enough blood to meet your body's needs. The BNP level in the blood increases when heart failure symptoms worsen and decreases when the heart failure condition improves or is stable. Normally, only a low amount of BNP is found in your blood; a higher BNP level correlates with more severe heart failure.
- Chest x-ray
  - A chest x-ray is a picture of the lungs and the position of the heart in the chest. This test determines the presence of lung disease, detects fluid

in your lungs, and detects any potential silent lung cancer. A CT of the chest may be necessary to provide more detailed pictures.

- Electrocardiogram (ECG)
  - The electrocardiogram shows the pattern of electrical impulses in your heart. Small pads (electrode leads) connected with wires are placed over different parts of your body. These leads noninvasively detect the rhythm and pattern of the electrical waves of your heart and convert it into lines on a sheet of paper for your doctor to interpret.
- Echocardiogram (Echo)
  - An echocardiogram is a noninvasive form of cardiac imaging (an ultrasound of the heart) that uses sound waves to examine the size, shape, and motion of all cardiac structures. The important structures that are seen include the four heart valves, the pumping function of the right and left ventricles (lower chambers), and the pericardial sac (the lining of the heart). This test is used to determine your ejection fraction (EF), which is a measurement of the percentage of blood that your heart ejects with each beat.
- MUGA
  - A MUGA is a noninvasive nuclear medicine picture test. Your vein is injected with a nonradioactive compound, and a special camera is placed over your chest while you are lying down, to measure the ability of your heart to pump blood. This test is specifically used to measure your ejection fraction.
- Exercise tolerance (treadmill) test
  - This noninvasive procedure monitors you and your heart's response to strenuous exercise. It is also known as a "stress test." You are connected to wires and electrode leads, just like when you have an electrocardiogram (ECG). Your monitored

walking on the treadmill functions as a "stress" to the heart and can measure your exercise tolerance and capacity.

- Pulmonary function test (PFT)
  - A pulmonary function test is a series of breathing tests that are performed on your lungs to measure their capacity and their ability to carry oxygen. This is done to detect any lung disease and to determine your ability to wean from the breathing ventilator after your transplant surgery.
- Noninvasive carotid artery Doppler studies
  - This is an ultrasound of the carotid (neck) arteries that looks for blockages in the arteries that supply blood to the brain, which is more common in patients who have atherosclerosis. If the carotid arteries have severe narrowing, this must be corrected before your transplant surgery.
- Abdominal ultrasound
  - An ultrasound of your belly is a painless test performed to rule out any gallbladder disease/stones and to assess for an abnormally enlarged abdominal aorta (aneurysm).
- Bone scan (DEXA scan)
  - A bone scan is used specifically to assess the risk of fracture by detecting osteoporosis, which is a thinning of the bones that can occur with aging. The scan takes approximately 10 minutes. Low-energy x-rays are passed through the bones to measure the mineral (calcium) content of the bones. Not all patients require this test.
- Skin tests
  - A skin test is performed to check for exposure to tuberculosis. A small needle is used on your arm to inject a serum in three different places. Your arm is then checked within 48 hours to look for a skin reaction. If the test reveals that you have

been exposed to tuberculosis, you will be treated with certain medications while waiting for your heart transplant.

- Urine tests
  - A routine urinalysis is sent to look for any type of urine infection. If needed, a 24-hour urine collection is done to further assess your kidney function.
- Mammogram/Pap smear
  - A gynecologic exam is performed on all women who have not had recent testing. It is important to undergo a comprehensive cancer screening as a part of your transplant evaluation.
- Prostate test
  - A simple prostate specific antigen (PSA) laboratory test is performed in men to exclude any silent prostate cancer. If necessary, a supplemental prostate exam may be required.
- Stool sample to detect blood
  - A simple stool sample test (a "stool guaiac card") is an easy way to check the stool for any hidden blood in the intestinal tract. Blood in the stool can possibly indicate a hidden colon cancer. If necessary, a colonoscopy may be required to more carefully exclude any potential colon cancer.
- Left heart catheterization and coronary angiogram
  - This is described in more detail in Question 74. A left heart catheterization allows your doctor to actually see how the blood flows through your heart and coronary arteries. When dye is injected into your coronary arteries to take an x-ray movie picture, it is called a coronary angiogram. This is the best way to evaluate the coronary arteries for any potential blockage problems. It is usually done through a small catheter (fine hollow tube) inserted into an artery on the side of your groin (the femoral artery).

- Right heart catheterization
  - This is described in more detail in Question 74. This invasive test is performed to measure the pressures inside the right side of your heart and to check for the presence of pulmonary hypertension (elevated pressure in the lungs). It is usually done through the right jugular vein on the side of the neck.
- Cardiopulmonary stress test (VO_2).
  - This is described in more detail in Question 76. This is a special type of exercise test that measures your combined heart and lung function and ability to use oxygen. You walk on a treadmill while attached to a special breathing monitor/apparatus.

74. What is a heart catheterization?

A heart catheterization is an invasive heart test performed by a cardiologist using your arteries or veins to obtain information about your heart and its function. It may involve a left heart catheterization, a right heart catheterization, or both.

Left Heart Catheterization and Coronary Angiogram

A left heart catheterization allows your doctor to actually see how the blood flows through your heart and coronary arteries. When dye is injected into your coronary arteries to take an x-ray movie picture, it is called a coronary angiogram. This is the best way to evaluate the coronary arteries for any potential blockage problems.

After carefully cleaning and sterilizing the area, a cardiologist inserts a catheter (a small, fine, hollow tube) into an artery on the side of your groin and uses an x-ray camera to guide the catheter up to your heart. From the tip of the catheter, the doctor can inject a small amount of dye into each coronary artery and take an x-ray movie picture of all your coronary arteries. These pictures show up on the monitor screens and are recorded digitally. Pictures of your heart's pumping function can also be obtained to measure your ejection fraction.

You are awake but sedated during this routine procedure, which takes approximately 1 hour. The procedure takes place in the cardiac catheterization laboratory, and you can go home several hours after the test is completed.

It is likely that you will have a left heart catheterization at some time before you undergo a heart transplant. After your transplant, you will also have this procedure as a part of your annual posttransplant check-up. A left heart catheterization is often accompanied by a right heart catheterization (see below).

Right Heart Catheterization

A right heart catheterization is an invasive test that is performed to measure the pressures inside the right side of your heart. It is done to check for the presence of pulmonary hypertension (elevated pressure in the lungs).

After carefully cleaning the side of your neck, a cardiologist inserts a small catheter (a fine, hollow tube) into the large vein on the side of your neck (the jugular vein). This special catheter has a soft inflatable balloon on the tip, known as a Swan-Ganz catheter or a pulmonary artery catheter. The tip of this catheter is then advanced into the right-sided chambers of the heart (atrium and ventricle) and then advanced out into the pulmonary artery, which is the main artery that leaves the heart and delivers blood to the lungs (this is why it is called a pulmonary artery catheter). The pressures in each of your heart chambers and in your lungs (pulmonary artery pressure) are carefully measured and recorded. These pressures are also known as your **hemodynamics**.

This test is performed before you are considered for a heart transplant. It is also scheduled periodically (usually every 6 months) while you are waiting on the transplant list to make sure no changes have occurred.

Some patients are so sick while waiting for a heart transplant that they require a long-term pulmonary artery catheterization, whereby the Swan-Ganz catheter is left in their neck until they receive a new heart. Their tenuous medical condition may require continual monitoring of their heart pressures to prevent their clinical status from deteriorating while they await a new heart. Because they are so sick, these patients have a preferred status on the heart transplant waiting list.

Hemodynamics

Pressures in each of your heart chambers and in your lungs (pulmonary artery pressure).

75. What is pulmonary hypertension? What is a vasoactive drug study?

A right heart catheterization is an important test that is performed to measure the pressures inside the right side of your heart. More importantly, it is done to check for the presence of pulmonary hypertension.

In patients who have severe heart failure, the pulmonary artery pressure (pressure in the lung arteries) can become elevated due to the chronic congestion in the heart and lungs. This is known as **pulmonary hypertension** and essentially is high blood pressure in the arteries that supply the lungs. The right heart catheterization (using a Swan-Ganz catheter) can precisely measure and record this pressure. These pressures are also referred to as your hemodynamics.

Pulmonary hypertension

High blood pressure in the arteries that supply the lungs.

If your right heart catheterization demonstrates pulmonary hypertension, the cardiologist may need to consider additional testing during your catheterization. This is referred to as a vasoactive drug study. If the pulmonary pressures are too high, special intravenous medications (**vasoactive drugs**) are given to try to lower the pulmonary pressures or to increase the forward pumping force of the heart (the cardiac output). They are called vasoactive because they typically work by acting on the blood vessels in the body, typically dilating (enlarging) them, which can act to lower the pressure in the arteries. This may reduce the pulmonary artery pressure and may increase the cardiac output of the heart.

These vasoactive medicines are given slowly according to a standardized administration protocol. At each stage of the protocol, careful measurements of the hemodynamics are repeated and measured. Usually, the pulmonary pressures eventually come down with escalating doses of the medicines, and the test may then be concluded. It the pressures do come down, then the person's pulmonary hypertension is deemed "reversible."

If a patient's pulmonary pressures do not decrease/improve with the special intravenous medicines during the drug study and still remain too high, their pulmonary hypertension is deemed to be "fixed" or "irreversible." This situation is a major concern, because when a patient develops fixed pulmonary hypertension, there is a significant risk that a new transplanted heart will not function properly in their chest, and the new heart may fail shortly after the transplantation. If this is the case, these patients may not be eligible to receive a heart transplant.

Vasoactive drugs

Medications given to try to lower the pulmonary pressures or to increase the forward pumping force of the heart (the cardiac output).

Fixed pulmonary hypertension is a contraindication to transplantation because of the high risk of posttransplant failure. While you are on the heart transplant waiting list, you will undergo periodic right heart catheterizations to exclude this type of pulmonary hypertension. If pulmonary hypertension is present, then a vasoactive drug study will be performed to demonstrate that it remains reversible. As long as it remains reversible, you are still eligible for a heart transplant.

76. What is a cardiopulmonary metabolic stress test?

A cardiopulmonary metabolic exercise stress test is also referred to as a CPX test or a VO_2-Max test. This is a special type of exercise test that measures your combined heart and lung function and your body's ability to use oxygen at rest and with exercise. You walk on a treadmill while attached to a special breathing monitor/apparatus. Sometimes a bicycle is used.

This special breathing apparatus is called a "metabolic cart," and it uses sophisticated technology that precisely quantifies your oxygen intake, carbon dioxide exhalation, your metabolic rate (your body's baseline energy expenditure without exercise), as well as your heart's and lung's ability to properly process and use oxygen while exercising.

Cardiopulmonary exercise testing provides important information in a patient who has heart failure. The "maximal oxygen consumption" is known as the "VO_2-Max" or the "MVO_2." The VO_2-Max is regulated by your heart function, and it reflects the maximum amount of oxygen that your heart can provide to your muscles during sustained activity. The VO_2-Max is the point at which your body cannot increase its intake of oxygen despite an increase in exercise intensity. This is quantified as a number.

Under normal circumstances a healthy body continues to increase oxygen intake and uptake as it increases its exercise intensity. Patients who have heart failure have decreased exercise capacity and a diminished ability to properly augment oxygen intake to meet increasing body demands. They have a lower VO_2-Max; a lower VO_2-Max number correlates with worse heart failure symptoms as well as a worsened overall prognosis. Studies have shown that the VO_2-Max is one of the strongest predictors of survival in patients with heart failure.

Because of this established correlation in heart failure patients, your maximal oxygen consumption number is considered as a part of your transplant evaluation. A healthy person should have a VO_2-Max of well over 25 mL/kg/min. In most transplant centers, a VO_2-Max score of less than 14 mL/kg/min qualifies you for a transplant. Of course, as with all of your pretransplant testing, your case is considered individually, but this is still an important component of your evaluation.

77. I also have kidney problems. Can more than one organ be transplanted at the same time?

Most patients who have heart failure also experience some degree of kidney problems during the course of their medical illness. The syndrome of heart failure involves a reduced forward pumping of blood out of the heart (reduced cardiac output). The reduced pumping function of the heart diminishes the amount of oxygen-rich blood that is delivered to the vital organs, especially the kidneys. A reduction in adequate blood flow to the kidneys can adversely affect how they function.

Additionally, some other medical conditions that often accompany heart failure, such as high blood pressure and diabetes, can contribute and directly impact the kidneys, which can further compound the problem and can cause additional weakening of the kidney function. Sometimes, the medicines that are used to treat heart failure can actually worsen kidney function, such as diuretics (water pills) or other heart medicines (ACE inhibitors, ARBs, or aldosterone antagonists).

If your kidneys do not function properly, several heart failure conditions may become worsened. If the filtering system of the kidney fails, wastes can accumulate, and certain electrolytes (like potassium) may become unregulated. Abnormal levels of these electrolytes can be dangerous to a weakened heart. It is not uncommon for patients with weakened kidneys to develop higher blood pressure, which may increase the workload to the tired heart. Also, the weakened kidney can have difficulty properly managing your fluid and water status, which can lead to worsened water retention, swelling, bloating, and worsened overall heart failure status.

It is clear that the heart and kidneys need to maintain a delicate balance and have a carefully entwined relationship. Any weakening in either condition adversely impacts the other's proper functioning. This is often referred to as the **cardiorenal syndrome** (or, the "heart-kidney" syndrome) and can make managing and treating both conditions simultaneously very difficult. Fortunately, for most heart failure patients, when their heart failure improves, so will their kidney function.

Cardiorenal syndrome

Syndrome in which any weakening in either condition adversely impacts the other's proper functioning, because the heart and kidneys need to maintain a delicate balance and have a carefully entwined relationship.

Sometimes, however, a patient may develop permanent kidney damage or kidney failure. If this is the case, newer techniques allow patients to be listed for both a heart and a kidney transplant at the same time. The need for combined organ transplantation does not elevate your status on the waiting list. The organs for a patient who requires combined organ transplantation come from a single organ donor, because they will already be properly matched to the recipient.

In other rare circumstances, if a patient has cirrhosis and is otherwise a good candidate for heart transplantation, a combined heart–liver transplantation may be considered. This depends on the level of experience at your individual transplant program.

PART THREE

Organ Allocation

Where does a donor heart come from?

How many heart transplants are performed each year in the United States?

How does the heart transplant waiting list work? How is it prioritized? Can I be on heart transplant waiting lists in more than one region?

More . . .

78. *How are heart transplant organs allocated?*

Globally, the need for organ transplantation continues to exceed the supply of donor organs. The transplant community is organized under a nationwide umbrella, called the **United Network for Organ Sharing (UNOS)**. UNOS is a private, nonprofit organization that matches available organ donors with those awaiting transplantation. UNOS is under contract with the U.S. Department of Health and Human Services to maintain the nation's organ transplant waiting list. UNOS guarantees that all persons who need a transplant have an equal opportunity to receive their organs, regardless of age, gender, race, social status, and so on.

There are 11 geographic UNOS regions in the country. These regions play a role in organ allocation, as organs are offered to sick patients within the same region in which they are donated before being offered to other parts of the country.

There are 58 **organ procurement organizations (OPOs)** in the United States. These are private, nonprofit organizations that coordinate the organ procurement in a designated service area, which may cover all or only part of a state. The OPO evaluates potential donors, discusses donation with potential donor family members, arranges for the surgical removal of donated organs, and arranges for the distribution of the organs according to national organ-sharing policies.

The allocation of an available donor heart is determined by a number of strict established criteria, specifically

- Blood type (A, B, AB, O types) compatibility
- Severity of illness (acuity) or medical urgency of the recipient, according to UNOS criteria ("UNOS status")

United Network for Organ Sharing (UNOS)

A private, nonprofit organization that matches available organ donors with those awaiting transplantation.

Organ procurement organization (OPO)

Private, nonprofit organizations in the United States that coordinate organ procurement in a designated service area, which may cover all or only part of a state.

- Body size compatibility
- The length of time a person has been on the waiting list

All this information is then entered into the UNOS computerized waiting list. When a heart becomes available, it is given to the best possible match, based on these strict established criteria. The race and gender of the donor have no bearing on the match.

During your transplant evaluation process, a test is performed to determine your blood type. This plays a role in determining a "donor match," or from which donors you can accept a heart (**Table 6**). In general, candidates on the list receive an identically matched blood group heart (as determined by ABO blood typing), regardless of the Rh factor (rhesus factor, the + or − sign that occurs after the blood type). Fortunately, matching the Rh factor does not seem to have any significant influence of the outcome of the transplant or the likelihood of rejection. Because some blood groups are more common than others, the amount of time on the waiting list may be influenced by your blood type as well as the blood type of any available donors.

Table 6   Acceptable Matches of Recipient and Donor Blood Types

Recipient Blood Type	Acceptable Donor Blood Type
O	O
A	O, A
B	O, B
AB	O, A, B, AB

79. Where does a donor heart come from?

Your new heart must come from someone who has been declared brain dead and whose family agrees to donate the organs. It is an anonymous gift. Brain death is a permanent condition usually due to a head injury from a car accident, gunshot wound, or a hemorrhage into the brain (like a stroke). It means that although the body is being kept alive by machines, the brain has no signs of life. Brain death is diagnosed by many different tests and is confirmed by two doctors who are not involved with the donor's care.

The donor's heart continues to beat independently and may be supported by intravenous medications in an intensive care unit (ICU). Breathing and respirations are maintained by a mechanical ventilator. Then, the donor is evaluated to determine if the organs are suitable for transplantation. The donor undergoes blood work similar to your pretransplant evaluation. Extensive predonation cardiac testing on the donor heart is also performed, such as an electrocardiogram, echocardiogram, and possibly a coronary angiogram and heart catheterization. These tests are done to ensure that the donor heart is suitable for transplantation.

All this information is then entered into the UNOS computerized waiting list. This waiting list ensures equal access and fair distribution of organs when they become available. When a heart becomes available, it is given to the best possible match, based on strict established criteria (blood type, body size, UNOS status, and length of time on the waiting list). The race and gender of the donor have no bearing on the match.

Many people who are waiting for transplantation have mixed feelings because they are aware that someone must die before an organ becomes available. It may help to know that many donor families feel a sense of peace knowing that some good has come from their loved one's tragic death.

80. How many heart transplants are performed each year in the United States?

At any given time over 3,000 people are on the national patient waiting list for a heart transplant. Only about 2,200 donor hearts become available for transplant each year. Interestingly, these figures have not changed significantly for nearly 20 years. There have been campaigns to raise awareness of the importance of organ donation, but these have not yielded any significant increase in the number of available heart transplant donors. This disparity means that some patients die waiting for a new heart.

Ultimately, as the technology of ventricular assist devices (VAD) improves and their usage becomes more widespread, there may be a significant increase in the utilization of this device. This potential increase in VAD use may help to bridge the gap between the numbers of needy heart failure patients on the waiting list and the numbers of available donor hearts.

81. How does the heart transplant waiting list work? How is it prioritized? Can I be on heart transplant waiting lists in more than one region?

Once you agree to the transplant process, you are placed on the heart transplant waiting list. Once listed, the wait can last from several days to several years. The waiting list is maintained by UNOS and is organized by several established factors that play a role in the timing of your eventual heart transplant. Blood type, medical acuity/urgency, body size, and number of days waiting on the transplant list are the factors considered.

Your blood type (ABO blood typing) plays a role in determining which available donors are eligible to donate to you (a "donor match"). In general, candidates on the list receive an identically matched blood group heart.

In addition to matching blood type, further blood testing is performed to determine if you have developed any antibodies to specific human antigens. Antibodies are produced by your immune system and develop in persons who have been exposed to human proteins that are not of their own genetic makeup. This can occur with blood transfusions or during a pregnancy. Your doctors perform what is called a **panel reactive antibody (PRA) test** when you are listed. If you have a high PRA, you will have to wait longer for a more compatible heart. A high PRA means that you are highly reactive to specific antigens ("sensitized") and that your doctors need to be more selective with the donor heart chosen for you to avoid acute rejection.

Finally, when a donor organ does become available, ABO blood typing is performed, and then the organ is offered to the patient in the region who has the most urgent medical need for the organ, based on his or her current health status (UNOS medical urgency status). There are three medical urgency status categories for patients waiting for a heart transplant.

Status 1A is the top of the UNOS waiting list. These patients are determined to be critically ill because they require mechanical or chemical support in the form of a breathing machine (ventilator), intraaortic balloon pump (catheter inserted in leg to help the heart pump), continuous intravenous infusions of powerful

Panel reactive antibody (PRA) test

A blood test performed before transplantation to determine if you have developed any antibodies to specific human antigens.

cardiac medications with a special catheter in their neck (called a Swan-Ganz catheter), and/or a newly implanted ventricular assist device (VAD). These patients are usually very sick in the intensive care unit and will die without a heart transplant.

The second UNOS group is referred to as status 1B. These patients may be in or out of the hospital and have continuous intravenous medications and/or a VAD longer than 30 days postoperatively from activation on the waiting list. Individuals with these types of support measures maintain status 1B even if discharged home with this type of treatment.

The last UNOS category is status 2. Most patients in this category are out of the hospital and stable. Their medical condition is carefully monitored and updated.

There are 11 geographic UNOS regions in the country. Organs are procured and distributed within each region. Organs are offered to sick patients within the same region in which they are donated before they are offered to other parts of the country. It is not common for a heart to be donated to a recipient outside of its own local region. Because of this regional allocation, each region has its own supply and demand for heart transplants. Thus regions with a larger supply of donor hearts and smaller demand of waiting patients have a shorter wait list time for a new heart.

The UNOS statutes do allow you to be on the heart transplant waiting list in more than one region ("multiple listing"). A candidate will not benefit from being listed by two transplant programs within the same local UNOS region, because all programs within a single region work from the same master list.

It is important to know that some transplant programs may have policies that prohibit multiple-listed patients. Others may set their own requirements or preconditions for multiple-listed candidates (for example, ability to come to the hospital within a certain amount of time if you are called for an organ offer).

If a patient chooses to be listed by more than one program in different UNOS regions, there are five other issues to consider in addition to the individual transplant program's policies as above.

1. Your insurance may not cover the cost of an additional evaluation or pay for a transplant outside of your local region.
2. The additional expenses of travel and lodging outside of your region often are not reimbursed.
3. No matter how sick you are or become, you must get to the outside region transplant center quickly, because organs become available on very short notice.
4. Most transplant programs require their recipients to stay in close proximity to their center for at least 1 month after the transplant to monitor recovery, assess for rejection, perform biopsies, and adjust transplant medications.
5. If you were to experience any major posttransplant complication, you must be able to return to your transplant center for specialized posttransplant care.

Remember, it is not possible to predict how well or sick you may be while waiting for your new heart transplant. Even though the waiting time may indeed be shorter at a program outside of your local region, it still may not be the *best overall* strategy to be listed and transplanted at a center farther from home.

PART FOUR

Preparing for Transplantation

Are there special diets for patients who have
congestive heart failure?

Am I allowed to exercise before my heart
transplantation?

After I am on the heart transplant waiting list,
how long will I have to wait to receive a new heart?
Will I have to wait in the hospital?

82. Are there special diets for patients who have congestive heart failure?

The good news is that there is a lot you can do to help your heart condition and to reduce your heart failure symptoms.

Good nutrition is important for patients who have heart failure. The most important thing you can do is to carefully restrict the salt (sodium chloride) in your diet. A high-salt diet can increase your blood pressure but, more importantly, can cause your body to retain water. This can cause swelling and worsened symptoms. You should limit your sodium intake to 2,000 milligrams (mg) per day. This is about the amount of salt in a teaspoon.

The first and easiest way to reduce your salt intake is take the salt shaker off the table. Keep it out of reach, or even throw it away. Use fresh vegetables and foods instead of canned or processed foods. Learn to read food labels to keep track of how much sodium you eat. A consultation with a registered dietitian may be helpful.

Observing a "heart-healthy" diet and avoiding overeating is a good idea. Increase the amount of fruits and vegetables you eat each day. Eliminate any fried foods or foods that are high in cholesterol. Reduce your intake of red meat, and increase the amount of "white" meat or fish in your diet. If you have diabetes, maintain a strict low-carbohydrate and low-sugar diet.

You may be told to limit your fluid intake to help prevent edema and water retention. This includes anything that is liquid at room temperature (such as soups, juices, popsicles, and ice cream). Measuring drinks in a measuring cup before you drink them may help you maintain your daily fluid goals. Other tips include chewing gum or sucking on hard candy or lemon wedges, only drinking when you are thirsty, and rinsing your mouth with water without swallowing it.

Be smart about alternative or herbal remedies. You may have heard about supplements and herbs that claim to help the heart or help heart failure symptoms. These claims are being studied but have not been medically proven. Keep in mind that "natural" does not mean "safe." Extracts, herbs, and other supplements can interact with your prescription medicines. Some over-the-counter products are not safe and can cause organ damage. If you want to try alternative or herbal treatments, be sure to discuss it with your doctor first.

83. Am I allowed to exercise before my heart transplantation?

Heart failure patients need to stay active. Severely restricting your physical activity is not a good idea, because it can reduce your stamina and further lower your exercise capacity. Your heart failure symptoms will likely improve if you stay as physically active as possible. Aerobic activities, such as walking, can help by exercising the heart and may allow it to get stronger. When you stay active, you may feel less tired and have fewer symptoms. It is a good idea to have a regular exercise schedule. By exercising regularly and keeping your body conditioned, you feel better and can exercise longer.

When you are exercising, it is important to pace yourself. If you can't hold a conversation during activity, you are pushing yourself too hard. Try to do activities that involve your family or friends. Be sure to know your limits, and understand that you will likely have both good days and bad days. During your activities you should be careful not to overexert yourself. Stop exercising if you feel chest pain or burning, severe breathlessness, a racing heartbeat, or lightheadedness/dizziness.

Although it is important to stay active, your body also needs rest. Regular periods of both rest and exercise should be scheduled into your day. Allowing extra rest during time periods of emotional stress or illness may be helpful. If you listen to your body, you know when it needs rest or activity.

84. After I am on the heart transplant waiting list, how long will I have to wait to receive a new heart? Will I have to wait in the hospital?

Once you have been accepted as a candidate for a heart transplant, the wait for a new heart begins. At any given time about 3,100 people are on the national patient waiting list for a new heart, but only about 2,200 donor hearts become available for transplantation each year.

The average waiting time for a donor heart is about 6 months, but the wait can be much shorter or much longer, depending on the availability of a heart. The wait can sometimes be for several years. In addition to organ availability, the duration of the waiting period can be influenced by your blood group and how sick you are.

Some patients may have a serious medical event (such as a stroke, severe infection, kidney failure, etc.) while waiting for a heart transplant. If these are temporary, the patient may be temporarily removed ("inactivated") from the active list of patients awaiting a transplant. After they recover from this medical event, they may be "reactivated" on the list and return to their same place on the waiting list (and will not lose credit for the time they have already accumulated). Rarely, if it is a very severe and permanent problem, that patient may then no longer be considered as a candidate for a heart transplant, and other options are then considered.

At least one-third of patients on the transplant list are too sick to be discharged from the hospital and must remain in the hospital until the transplant is performed. Of course, these patients are given the highest priority, because some of them require intensive care unit monitoring and powerful intravenous cardiac medications or mechanical heart pumps (VADs) to keep them alive. That being said, over 50% of patients on the waiting list are at home when they are called to receive their heart transplant.

If at all possible, every effort is made to improve a patient's condition so that they can enjoy time at home while they wait for a new heart. To get some patients home for the long wait, a continuous infusion of special intravenous heart medication (dobutamine or milrinone) may be instituted, administered by a long-term intravenous (IV) line from a portable medicine infusion pack. As discussed earlier, some patients go home with a special heart pump (ventricular assist device).

PART FIVE

Surgery

How long will the heart transplantation surgery take?
How long will I need to be in the hospital after my
heart transplant?

What complications can happen
after my heart transplant?

85. How long will the heart transplantation surgery take? How long will I need to be in the hospital after my heart transplant?

For each heart transplant performed, there is a primary recipient and a backup recipient. If for some reason the primary recipient cannot receive the heart, the heart then goes to the backup. After you are notified at home or by pager about a donor heart transplant, it is typically several hours before you are taken to the operating room, so you do not need to rush.

While you are being prepared for your surgery, another team of surgeons is retrieving the heart from the organ donor ("procuring"). They are making sure that the donor heart is a healthy heart for you to receive. After the heart is removed from the donor, there is a 4-hour window in which it needs to be transplanted into you. Your wait, however, is likely to be longer than this.

After it is removed, the donor heart is cooled and placed in a special solution for preservation until it is ready to be transplanted. During the operation you are placed on a heart–lung machine ("cardiopulmonary bypass"). This machine is hooked up to your arteries and veins and allows your body to receive vital oxygen and nutrients from the blood even though the heart is being operated on.

After you receive general anesthesia and are asleep, the cardiothoracic surgeon makes an incision in your breastbone (sternum). The surgeon then removes your diseased heart, except for the back walls of the atria (the heart's upper chambers). The backs of the atria on the new heart are then opened, and the new heart is sewn into place. The surgeon then connects the major blood vessels, allowing blood to flow through the heart and lungs. As the transplanted heart warms up and blood flow is restored, it starts beating. An initial electric shock may be needed to help it restart the heartbeat. You are then weaned off the bypass machine with the help of your new heart.

It is a complicated operation that can last from 4 to 10 hours. After surgery you are transferred to the cardiothoracic intensive care unit to begin your recovery process.

How quickly you recover after your heart transplant depends on your age, overall health, and response to the transplant. Most patients are up and about within a few days after the surgery. If there are no signs of acute rejection, you can go home within 1 to 2 weeks after your transplant.

86. What complications can happen after my heart transplant?

It is important to remember that transplantation is a serious surgery and does still involve important risks. As with any major operation, there is a risk of both short-term and long-term complications. The most frequent cause of death in the first month after transplant is **primary graft dysfunction**. This occurs when the transplanted heart fails for unknown reasons and isn't able to function. This requires urgent retransplantation or the patient will die. Up to 5% of patients do not survive 30 days after their transplant.

According to recent data, however, most patients (approximately 88%) are alive and well after the first year of their new transplant. Rejection and infection are the most common and serious complications after transplantation, especially during that first year. Because

Primary graft dysfunction

Occurs when the transplanted heart fails for unknown reasons and isn't able to function, requiring urgent retransplantation to avoid patient death.

183

of the risk of rejection, you need very careful monitoring and frequent heart muscle biopsies (endomyocardial biopsy). Due to improvements in immunosuppressant medications and diagnostic testing, the rate of post-transplant rejection is decreasing. The prevention, early detection, and treatment of any infection are also crucially important to keeping both you and your new heart healthy.

Over the long term there are many other important health conditions that may develop in patients who have received a heart transplant; these usually occur several years after your transplant. Immunosuppressant medications (antirejection medicines) increase the long-term risk of infections, but these infections can be treated. Your doctors also monitor you carefully for some of the medical problems that can develop after your transplant, specifically high blood pressure, diabetes mellitus, high cholesterol, osteoporosis, kidney disease, cataracts, and cancer.

Immunosuppressant medications can also raise the risk of getting certain types of cancer, especially blood cancer (lymphoma) and skin cancer. Although lymphoma can rarely be fatal, your doctor can lower the risk of developing this by reducing the dosage of your antirejection medicines. About 1 in every 10 transplant patients develops some form of cancer after their heart transplant. Other common forms of cancer (lung, colon, breast, etc.) are not more common in heart transplant patients than they are in the general population.

PART SIX

After Transplantation

Will I be able to return to work after my
heart transplantation?

What is an endomyocardial biopsy?
How often will I need one?

How long do patients live after a heart transplant?

87. Will I be able to return to work after my heart transplantation?

In the days immediately after your transplant, you can expect to be tired. Heart transplantation is a major operation. However, you will begin to feel better and stronger each day.

After your heart transplant, you can and should exercise. Your heart will react differently to physical activity after your transplant. This is because the nerves that connected your original heart to your nervous system were cut during the surgery ("denervated heart"). Because these nerves will not heal, your heart cannot respond immediately to exercise, sudden movement, or emotional stress, like fear. It does react, but not nearly as fast. It may take some time to get used to how your new heart responds. Starting an exercise program expedites your recovery and helps you feel better faster.

After you are released from the hospital, you are closely monitored for 3 to 6 months. You cannot drive for a few months. During the first few months your immune system is very suppressed due to your antirejection medications. You need to observe special precautions to reduce your risk of infection. You may need to wear a mask when out in public, and you should avoid large crowds.

You can expect to return to a healthy, active life within 3 to 6 months after your heart transplant. Many patients are then able to resume recreational activities and return back to work, either part time or full time, within a few months. Exercise and a healthy diet are essential to your successful recovery. Nearly 85% of patients return to work or other activities they previously enjoyed.

88. What is an endomyocardial biopsy? How often will I need one?

Rejection is the most common and serious complication after heart transplantation, especially during the first year. Because of the risk of rejection you need very careful monitoring and frequent heart muscle biopsies (**endomyocardial biopsy**). Rejection must be detected and treated quickly to prevent damage to the transplanted heart.

Endomyocardial biopsy

Heart muscle biopsy after transplantation to monitor for rejection.

The follow-up and testing schedule after a transplant is fairly intense for the first few months. Half of all possible rejections occur in the first 6 weeks, and most happen within the first 6 months of surgery.

Heart transplant recipients are carefully monitored for signs of rejection. The best method of checking your new heart for any signs of rejection is to perform a heart muscle biopsy (endomyocardial biopsy). This procedure is performed in the cardiac catheterization laboratory. It is usually an outpatient procedure that takes less than 1 hour to perform; you can return home after the procedure. Biopsies are scheduled routinely by your transplant team but may also be done if you develop any new symptoms that might suggest possible rejection.

Under local anesthetic a small catheter (a fine, hollow tube) is introduced through a vein in the neck and is passed into the heart, using an x-ray machine for guidance. This technique is very similar to a right heart catheterization procedure. At the tip of the catheter is a bioptome, which is a tiny tweezer-like instrument that is used to snip off a very small piece of heart muscle tissue. You will not feel any pain from this procedure but may feel some slight pressure. Then, these very small specimens of heart muscle tissue (endomy-ocardium) are taken from the heart and withdrawn through the catheter. A small bandage is placed on the site where the doctor inserted the catheter into your neck vein.

These biopsies are examined under the microscope for any signs of damage to the heart. If the biopsy shows any signs of damage to the heart cells due to rejection, the dose and kind of your immunosuppressant medications may be changed to further suppress the rejection.

You need to undergo periodic biopsies to make certain that even the earliest signs of rejection are detected. In the weeks after transplantation the cardiac biopsies occur more frequently; as time goes on these biopsies become less frequent. For each transplant recipient, depending on the biopsy results, the biopsy schedule varies.

Endomyocardial biopsies are usually scheduled weekly for the first 4 weeks after transplant and then every other week for about 1 to 2 months. After that, biopsies usually occur every 1 to 3 months for the first year and then once per year thereafter. After your yearly exam and biopsy, the schedule of biopsies depends on your transplant doctor and the amount of rejection detected, if any.

89. How long do patients live after a heart transplant?

For those people who are fortunate enough to receive a heart transplant, the long-term outlook is now very good indeed. How long you live after a transplant depends on many factors, including age, general health, and response to the heart transplant.

Recent data suggest that the 1-year survival after transplant is 88%, about 75% are alive after 5 years, and over 50% are alive after 10 years. The average length of survival is over 9 years.

The quality of life is usually good, especially if the side effects of the immunosuppressant medications can be kept to a minimum.

PART SEVEN

Complications

What is transplant rejection? How is it detected?
How is it treated?

Can my new transplanted heart develop "blockages?"
What is cardiac allograph vasculopathy (CAV)?

90. What is transplant rejection? How is it detected? How is it treated?

Your body possesses a natural defense mechanism, called the immune system, that under normal circumstances acts to protect you against injury due to such things as infection and trauma. After your transplant, the immune system perceives the transplanted heart as a "foreign" material and attempts to destroy it. If the immune system is able to attack the transplanted heart, it is called rejection. To suppress this response, you must take certain antirejection drugs (immunosuppressant medications) for life.

Rejection must be detected and treated quickly to prevent damage to the transplanted heart. It is not possible to predict who rejects, how frequently, or how severely, but almost all patients experience one or more rejection episodes at some time after their heart transplant. Your transplant doctors will teach you how to watch carefully for any symptoms of rejection.

Potential symptoms of heart transplant rejection are

- Sudden unexplained fatigue
- Decreased exercise tolerance
- Worsened shortness of breath
- Fluid retention, swollen ankles, feeling bloated
- Recurrence of your previous heart failure symptoms
- Palpitations or an irregular heartbeat
- Increased or high blood pressure
- Fever
- Flu-like symptoms or malaise

Acute transplant rejection is the leading cause of death in the first month after transplantation. It is essential to detect and treat acute rejection as early as possible, preferably before the injury is sufficient to cause symptoms to appear. For this reason you will undergo a series of routine examinations and testing at set intervals. These tests are carried out frequently during the first 6 months after your transplant, because this is when rejection most commonly occurs. Half of all possible rejections occur in the first 6 weeks, and most happen within the first 6 months of surgery.

The best method of checking your new heart to detect any signs of rejection is to perform a heart muscle biopsy (endomyocardial biopsy), described in Question 88. Small specimens of heart muscle tissue (endomyocardium) are taken from the heart and are examined under the microscope for any signs of damage to the heart.

Another way to check the transplanted heart for rejection is to perform an echocardiogram (cardiac ultrasound) to assess the pumping function of the heart. A heart that is experiencing some rejection may show signs of temporary weakening.

The treatment of rejection depends on the severity of the rejection, as determined by biopsy results and how well you are doing clinically. Most episodes of rejection are mild and can be treated at home with intravenous steroids and/or adjustment of your immunosuppressant medications. If there is evidence of more severe rejection, you may be admitted to the hospital for close monitoring and to receive other intravenous antirejection medicines.

91. Can my new transplanted heart develop blockages? What is cardiac allograph vasculopathy?

Although acute rejection of your new heart is rare after the first 6 months, the body may continue to attack the new heart. Narrowing in the coronary arteries (or blockages) of your transplanted heart can occur after a transplant and is sometimes called chronic rejection.

This chronic rejection is called cardiac allograph vasculopathy, which means literally "heart transplant blood vessel abnormality." It can occur anytime after a transplant but is not typically seen until several years after transplantation.

This type of coronary artery disease is different from the commonly seen fatty cholesterol plaques that occur in nontransplanted hearts with atherosclerosis (the kind you may have experienced before your transplant). Transplant allograph vasculopathy is mediated by the immune system. It causes a diffuse, smooth, widespread narrowing of all the coronary arteries. Unlike coronary arteries with atherosclerosis, cardiac allograph vasculopathy cannot be fixed by balloon angioplasty or coronary artery stenting.

To monitor for this condition, you undergo a cardiac catheterization and coronary angiogram at your first year anniversary. This is compared with a noninvasive imaging stress test of your heart (either ultrasound or nuclear medicine). Thereafter a noninvasive imaging stress test is performed annually. If these tests show any abnormality, a follow-up coronary angiogram may be arranged.

Treatment of posttransplant vasculopathy is very difficult, so prevention is the key. After a transplant you must follow a heart-healthy lifestyle and take medicines to help lessen the risk of vasculopathy and future coronary artery disease. Keeping both your cholesterol and blood pressure under tight control is especially important.

Medications

Why are immunosuppressive drugs necessary?

What are the immunosuppressive drugs?

I thought I'd be able to stop many of the medications I took before the transplant. Why am I still taking so many medications?

More . . .

92. Why are immunosuppressive drugs necessary?

Antirejection medications (immunosuppressants) are prescribed to help your immune system accept your new organ. Your transplant team may prescribe any of several antirejection medications: cyclosporine, tacrolimus, sirolimus, prednisone, mycophenolate, azathioprine, and basiliximab or Daclizumab. Some are taken in pill form every day; others are administered intravenously. As long as you have a functioning transplanted organ, you will take one or more antirejection medications for the rest of your life. Following the dosing schedule determined by your transplant team is essential to your well-being. Your transplant team determines the appropriate medications for you. You may be asked to participate in a self-medication program while you are in the hospital. By taking responsibility for your own medications in the hospital while under the supervision of a nurse, you can make the transition to home less stressful. Remember, *taking your medications is your responsibility.*

93. What are the immunosuppressive drugs?

Immunosuppressive drugs decrease the function of your immune system so that your immune system does not react to (that is, reject) the new organ. Without immunosuppressive drugs the immune system would recognize the new organ as foreign and attack it.

The following includes the commonly prescribed immunosuppressive agents and their side effects. After transplantation you will be prescribed several, but not all, of these medications.

Tacrolimus

Tacrolimus (also called Prograf, FK-506) is a primary immunosuppressive agent and, like cyclosporine, a calcineurin inhibitor. It is newer than cyclosporine and was approved for use in the United States in 1995. Tacrolimus is never used in conjunction with cyclosporine.

Notes About Tacrolimus

- You should not stop taking tacrolimus or change the dose or the time at which you take it unless your transplant team instructs you to do so.
- Tacrolimus should be taken in the morning and at night, about 12 hours apart.
- The amount of tacrolimus in your blood is monitored by blood tests. Do not take tacrolimus on the day you are having blood tests done until after the blood is drawn.
- Always take the correct dose of tacrolimus after your blood has been drawn.
- Tacrolimus may interact with some commonly used medications, such as antibiotics and high blood pressure medications. It is important that you check with the transplant team before starting any new medications.

Possible Side Effects

Headaches; nausea; diarrhea; stomach cramps; hand tremors or shaking; high blood sugar; high blood potassium; abnormal kidney function; hair loss; sleep disturbances; numbness and tingling in hands, feet, and mouth; decreased ability of the body to fight infection; increased risk of certain types of cancer, such as skin cancer, cervical cancer, and rarely lymphoma (lymph node cancer).

Cyclosporine

Cyclosporine (also called Neoral, Sandimmune, SangCya, Gengraf, Eon) is a primary immunosuppressive agent that is classified as a calcineurin inhibitor. This drug has been in use to prevent rejection in transplant recipients for more than 30 years.

Notes About Cyclosporine

- You should not stop taking cyclosporine or change the dose or the time at which you take it unless your transplant team instructs you to do so.
- Cyclosporine should be taken in the morning and at night, about 12 hours apart. Some patients need only one dose daily.
- The amount of cyclosporine in your blood is monitored by blood tests. Do not take cyclosporine on the day you are having blood tests until after the blood is drawn.
- Always take the correct dose of cyclosporine after your blood has been drawn.
- Cyclosporine may interact with some commonly used medications, such as antibiotics and high blood pressure medications. It is very important that you check with the transplant team before starting any new medications, especially antibiotics.

Possible Side Effects

Hand tremors or shaking; numbness or tingling in the hands, feet, mouth, or lips; decreased ability of the body to fight infection; abnormal kidney function tests; high blood pressure; swollen gums; hair growth; runny nose; high cholesterol; upset stomach; headache; increased risk of certain types of cancer, such as skin cancer, cervical cancer, and rarely lymphoma (lymph node cancer).

Sirolimus

Sirolimus (Rapamune, rapamycin) is another immunosuppressant that is similar in chemical structure to tacrolimus.

It does not cause kidney dysfunction but cannot be used immediately after transplantation because it delays healing of the surgical wound and rarely causes blood clots in the artery leading to the liver. Sirolimus is sometimes used several months or years after transplantation in patients who are at risk of kidney failure. It can be used in combination with low doses of cyclosporine or tacrolimus.

Notes About Sirolimus
- Take sirolimus 4 hours after cyclosporine or tacrolimus.
- Sirolimus comes in liquid and pill form. The liquid can be mixed only with water or orange juice and must be placed in a glass or plastic container.
- Sirolimus comes in a multidose bottle or single-dose foil pouches.
- Sirolimus liquid should be kept refrigerated.

Possible Side Effects
Elevated cholesterol and triglycerides, high blood pressure, rash, acne, anemia, joint pain, low potassium, low white blood cells, low platelets, anemia, diarrhea.

Prednisone
Prednisone (Deltasone, Orasone) is an immunosuppressant and anti-inflammatory medication. Although this drug is associated with many side effects, it remains an essential part of most posttransplant immunosuppressive regimens. You will receive your first dose of prednisone intravenously during the transplant operation.

Notes About Prednisone
- Do not stop taking prednisone or change the dose or the time at which you take it unless your transplant team instructs you to do so. A sudden discontinuation of prednisone can result in a severe illness called adrenal insufficiency.

- Always take prednisone with food or milk.
- If you have an episode of rejection, you may be instructed to take higher doses of prednisone.

Possible Side Effects

Increased appetite, acne, bruising, muscle weakness (especially in the upper legs and arms), stomach irritation, increased body and facial hair, mood change, decreased ability of the body to fight infections, high blood sugar, visual changes, delayed wound healing, softening of bones (osteoporosis), fluid and salt retention, anxiety, cataracts, glaucoma, night sweats, increased risk of certain cancers, menstrual irregularity.

Mycophenolate

Mycophenolate or mycophenolic acid (CellCept, Myfortic) belongs to a class of medications called antiproliferative drugs. These drugs are typically used in addition to a primary agent such as a calcineurin inhibitor.

Notes About Mycophenolate

- Do not stop taking mycophenolate mofetil or change the dose or the time at which you take it unless your transplant team instructs you to do so.
- Always swallow the capsules whole. Do not crush them, chew them, or open them.
- If a capsule comes apart, do not inhale the powder and do not let the powder touch your skin. If the powder touches your skin, wash it thoroughly with soap and water. If the powder comes in contact with your eyes, rinse them well with water.
- Do not take mycophenolate mofetil with antacids that contain magnesium or aluminum, such as Mylanta.
- Stomach cramps, nausea, and diarrhea may be controlled by spreading the dosage of mycophenolate mofetil over the course of the day. Ask your transplant

team if this is an option for you. Do not make any changes in your medication schedule before talking with them.

- You will have regular blood tests to monitor the effects of mycophenolate mofetil on your white blood cell count.
- Take mycophenolate mofetil 2 hours after cyclosporine or tacrolimus.
- Do not become pregnant or father a child while taking mycophenolate mofetil.

Possible Side Effects

Nausea; vomiting; diarrhea; stomach cramps; gas; decrease in appetite; decreased ability of the body to fight infection; increased risk of certain types of cancers, such as skin cancer, cervical cancer, and lymphoma (lymph node cancer).

Azathioprine

Azathioprine (Imuran) is an antiproliferative agent that is similar to mycophenolate. The two drugs are never used together.

Notes About Azathioprine

- Do not stop taking azathioprine or change the dose or the time at which you take it unless your transplant team instructs you to do so.
- You will have regular blood tests to monitor the effects of azathioprine on your white blood cell count.
- Do not take allopurinol (Zyloprim) for gout while taking azathioprine without discussing this issue with the transplant team.
- Women should avoid pregnancy while taking azathioprine. Contact your transplant team if you do become pregnant.

Possible Side Effects

Decreased ability of the body to fight infection; abnormal liver function tests (very rare); mouth sores; thinning hair; nausea; vomiting; bruising; increased risk of certain cancers, such as skin cancer, cervical cancer, and lymphoma (lymph node cancer).

Basiliximab

Basiliximab (Simulect) is a monoclonal antibody directed against parts of the immune system that cause acute rejection.

Notes About Basiliximab

- Basiliximab is used to prevent (but not to treat) episodes of acute rejection.
- Basiliximab can only be given intravenously.
- The first dose is usually administered in the operating room during the transplant operation.
- A second dose of basiliximab is given intravenously 4 days after the operation.

Possible Side Effects

Acne, constipation, nausea, diarrhea, headache, heartburn, trouble sleeping, weight gain, excessive hair growth, muscle or joint pain.

Daclizumab

Daclizumab (Zenapax) is a monoclonal antibody directed against parts of the immune system that cause acute rejection.

Notes About Daclizumab

- Daclizumab is used to prevent (but not to treat) episodes of acute rejection.
- Daclizumab can only be given intravenously.

- The first dose is usually administered in the operating room during the transplant operation.
- A second dose of Daclizumab is given intravenously 4 days after the operation.

Possible Side Effects

Chest pain, coughing, dizziness, fever, nausea, rapid heart rate, shortness of breath, swelling of the feet or lower legs, trembling or shaking of the hands or feet, vomiting, weakness.

94. Will I ever come off my immunosuppressive drugs?

Much of the success of organ transplantation can be attributed to improvements in the immunosuppressive drugs prescribed after the surgery. When the only drugs available were prednisone and azathioprine, the rejection rates and risk of graft loss were very high. Long-term survival was unusual. With the introduction of cyclosporine, however, patient survival increased almost immediately. The availability of even more drugs has since expanded the choices for safe and effective immunosuppression. Unfortunately, current immunosuppressive medications have a number of undesirable side effects (see Question 93).

Now that rejection has become a rare and controllable phenomenon, researchers are trying to determine the lowest amount of immunosuppression to prevent rejection and graft loss while at the same time minimizing the drugs' side effects. The advent of powerful primary agents, such as tacrolimus and sirolimus, has allowed us to decrease the overall number of drugs needed in one individual for adequate immunosuppression. The agent most commonly targeted for reduction has been prednisone—the drug with the most frequent and problematic side effects. The reduction in the use of prednisone has decreased the frequency of elevated blood sugars, osteoporosis, weight gain, and edema after transplantation. Many patients with no prior episodes of acute or chronic rejection, adequate kidney function, and acceptable liver and heart function tests are able to stop taking prednisone altogether. With the addition of mycophenolate to the primary agent, even patients with a history of mild rejection may be candidates to stop prednisone therapy.

A small number of reports from transplant centers have indicated that all immunosuppressive drugs may be stopped in a select group of transplant recipients. These reports emphasize the "success stories" and de-emphasize the failures and their outcomes—rejection, graft loss, retransplantation, or death. The difficulty arises in choosing the appropriate patient for total drug withdrawal. At this time we do not have any blood tests or markers that can reliably identify the best patients for removal of immunosuppression. Because the risks are so high (for example, graft loss), most transplant programs do not entertain the possibility of total immunosuppression withdrawal.

95. I thought I'd be able to stop many of the medications I took before the transplant. Why am I still taking so many medications?

You may be able to stop many of the medications you were taking before your transplant. Because of the multitude of risks and side effects caused by the immunosuppressive drugs, however, you need to take additional medications to minimize their risks and control the side effects. The immunosuppressive drugs decrease the function of your immune system. As a result, common viruses and bacteria, which are typically kept at bay by the intact immune system, may now cause serious infections. These potential infections include cytomegalovirus (CMV) and *Pneumocystis carinii* pneumonia (PCP).

CMV is a common virus that is similar to infectious mononucleosis. It may cause no symptoms or perhaps a febrile illness. When the immune system is intact, you can get CMV only once. However, in the immunosuppressed patient the virus can reemerge and cause inflammation in the new liver, kidney problems, pneumonia, and blood problems. *Pneumocystis carinii* infection usually causes pneumonia if it occurs in transplant recipients. Because these infections can be devastating or even fatal after transplantation, medications are prescribed to significantly reduce the risk of occurrence. As time goes by after transplantation, many of these preventive medications can be stopped as the degree of immunosuppression required to prevent rejection decreases.

Anti-Infection Medications (Antibacterials)

Antibiotics

Medications prescribed to prevent and treat bacterial infections.

Antibacterials (also called **antibiotics**) are prescribed to prevent and treat bacterial infections. Because antirejection medications can weaken your immune system, you are more at risk for the development of an infection, especially in your urinary tract or lungs. Antibiotics may be prescribed to decrease your chances of developing an infection and are definitely prescribed if an infection develops. Several antibiotics are commonly prescribed, including trimethoprim-sulfamethoxazole, levofloxacin, and ciprofloxacin.

Trimethoprim-sulfamethoxazole (TMP-SMZ, Bactrim, Cotrim, Septra) is prescribed to prevent PCP.

Notes About Trimethoprim-Sulfamethoxazole

- TMP-SMZ is available as a pill or a liquid.
- Take TMP-SMZ with 8 ounces of water.
- Do not take TMP-SMZ if you are allergic to sulfa.
- TMP-SMZ may be used to treat a urinary tract infection or pneumonia.
- Tell your transplant team if you become pregnant while taking TMP-SMZ.

Possible Side Effects

Low white blood cell count, nausea, vomiting, rash, itching, loss of appetite, abnormal kidney function tests.

Levofloxacin (Levaquin) and ciprofloxacin (Cipro) are antibiotics with many uses. They are effective therapy for some types of pneumonia (but not PCP), urinary tract infections, and bacterial cholangitis (infection of the bile ducts). Levofloxacin and ciprofloxacin are typically not used as preventive medicine but rather as a treatment.

Notes About Levofloxacin and Ciprofloxacin

- Drink a lot of fluids when taking levofloxacin or ciprofloxacin.
- Tell your transplant team if you have hives, a skin rash, or ringing in your ears.
- If you also are taking an antacid, do not take it within 2 hours of ciprofloxacin or levofloxacin.

Possible Side Effects

Upset stomach, diarrhea, nausea, vomiting, low blood sugar.

Antifungal Medications

Antifungal medications are prescribed to prevent and treat infections that are caused by fungus or yeast.

These include infections in the mouth (also called thrush), vagina (yeast infections), skin (jock itch, athlete's foot), blood, or lungs. There are several commonly prescribed antifungal medicines, including Mycostatin, clotrimazole, ketoconazole, and fluconazole.

Mycostatin (nystatin) is an antifungal medication primarily used to prevent thrush from developing in the mouth. It also comes in a powder to treat fungal skin infections like athlete's foot.

Notes About Mycostatin
- Mycostatin is a mouthwash that prevents or treats infections in your mouth.
- Mycostatin should be taken after meals and at bedtime.
- Make sure you do not have anything in your mouth before taking Mycostatin.
- Mycostatin is swished around in your mouth for a few minutes and then is swallowed.
- You should not eat or drink anything for 15 to 20 minutes after taking this medicine.
- Take good care of your mouth by brushing and flossing your teeth regularly.

Possible Side Effects
Nausea.

Clotrimazole (Mycelex) is an alternative to Mycostatin to prevent thrush.

Notes About Clotrimazole
- Clotrimazole is a lozenge that prevents or treats mouth infections.
- Clotrimazole should be taken after meals and at bedtime.

- You should let the lozenge dissolve in your mouth over a period of 15 minutes.
- Do not chew the lozenges or swallow them whole.

Possible Side Effects

Nausea, vomiting.

Ketoconazole (Nizoral) is another antifungal medication.

Notes About Ketoconazole

- Ketoconazole is a pill that should always be taken with food.
- Do not drink alcoholic beverages when taking ketoconazole.
- Antacids and acid blockers, such as Pepcid, Tagamet, or Zantac, should not be taken for at least 2 hours after taking ketoconazole.
- Call your doctor if you have a rash, itching, dark urine, pale stools, yellow skin, or sores in your mouth.
- Ketoconazole can affect the levels of cyclosporine, sirolimus, or tacrolimus found in your blood.
- Do not stop taking ketoconazole or change the dose or the time at which you take it unless your transplant team instructs you to do so, because such a change could have a serious effect on your cyclosporine or tacrolimus blood levels.

Possible Side Effects

Diarrhea, nausea, vomiting, impotence, menstrual irregularity, dizziness.

Fluconazole (Diflucan) is an antifungal with many uses. It can be used to treat known fungal infections and is often prescribed to prevent fungal infections.

Notes About Fluconazole

- Fluconazole can affect the amount of cyclosporine or tacrolimus found in your blood.

Medications

- Do not stop taking fluconazole or change the dose or the time at which you take it unless your transplant team instructs you to do so, because such a change could have a serious effect on your cyclosporine, sirolimus, or tacrolimus blood levels.

Possible Side Effects

Nausea, vomiting, diarrhea.

Antiviral Medications

Antiviral medications are prescribed to reduce the chance of specific viral infections, such as CMV and herpes, occurring after your transplant. You are at risk of developing these infections if you or your donor has had them at any time before transplantation. Antiviral medicines include valganciclovir, ganciclovir, and acyclovir.

Valganciclovir (Valcyte) and ganciclovir (Cytovene) are antiviral agents effective against the herpes viruses. These viruses include herpes simplex, CMV, and varicella (chickenpox).

Notes About Valganciclovir and Ganciclovir

- Do not stop taking valganciclovir or ganciclovir or change the dose or the time at which you take it unless your transplant team instructs you to do so.
- Valganciclovir and ganciclovir can be given in pill form or intravenously (in the vein).
- Call your transplant team if you have a skin rash, sore throat, fever, chills, or pain.

Possible Side Effects

Fever, rash, headache, abnormal kidney function tests, increased risk of infection, fatigue, diarrhea, nausea, vomiting.

Acyclovir (Zovirax) is occasionally used to prevent or treat herpes infections or varicella.

Notes About Acyclovir

- Do not become pregnant or father a child while you are taking acyclovir.
- Do not stop taking acyclovir or change the dose or the time at which you take it unless your transplant team instructs you to do so.
- If you are taking acyclovir for herpes simplex infection of the mouth or genitals, avoid kissing and sex if you have open sores.

Possible Side Effects

Nausea, vomiting, diarrhea, abnormal kidney function tests, rash, headache.

Medicines That Protect Your Digestive System

Two types of medicines that protect your digestive system are acid blockers and antacids. These agents are often necessary after transplantation to prevent stress ulcers in the stomach and gastroesophageal reflux disease (GERD) or heartburn symptoms.

Histamine-2 (H_2) acid blockers decrease the amount of acid produced by your stomach. They are used to prevent and treat ulcers. The most commonly used H_2 acid blockers are cimetidine (Tagamet), ranitidine (Zantac), famotidine (Pepcid), and nizatidine (Axid). These drugs are now available over the counter, but your transplant physician may want you to take prescription-strength doses.

Notes About Histamine-2 Acid Blockers

- Do not take an acid blocker at the same time you take fluconazole, ketoconazole, or another antacid.
- Take your acid blocker before meals.
- Your doctor will prescribe an acid blocker based on your needs.

Possible Side Effects

Diarrhea, constipation, nausea, gas, headache, dizziness.

Proton pump inhibitors block the formation of gastric acid in the stomach by inhibiting the activity at the surface where secretions are produced. The most commonly used proton pump inhibitors are omeprazole (Prilosec), lansoprazole (Prevacid), esomeprazole (Nexium), pantoprazole (Protonix), and rabeprazole (Aciphex). They are very well tolerated and extremely effective in treating ulcers and heartburn.

Notes About Proton Pump Inhibitors
- Swallow capsules whole. Do not open or crush them.

Possible Side Effects

Headache, diarrhea, abdominal pain.

High Blood Pressure Medications (Antihypertensives)

People who take high blood pressure medications before surgery are likely to continue to need those medications to lower their blood pressure after surgery. In addition, some people who had normal blood pressure before surgery may have high blood pressure after a transplant. Both cyclosporine and tacrolimus cause hypertension in about 70% of people who take them. The most commonly prescribed medicines for high blood pressure include diltiazem (Cardizem, Cartia, Dilacor, Tiazac), enalapril (Vasotec), lisinopril (Zestril), nifedipine (Procardia, Adalat), atenolol (Tenormin), and metoprolol (Lopressor).

Notes About Antihypertensive Medications
- You may be advised to follow a low-sodium diet if you have or develop high blood pressure.

- Some high blood pressure medications can affect your cyclosporine or tacrolimus blood levels. Check with your transplant team before starting or stopping any high blood pressure medication.

Possible Side Effects

Dizziness and lightheadedness for the first few days, fatigue, nausea, loss of appetite, headache, rash, dry cough, swelling in the feet, slow pulse, high potassium levels, kidney dysfunction.

Low Blood Pressure Medications

If your blood pressure is too low, your doctor may prescribe medicine to raise it. The medicine most commonly prescribed for low blood pressure is fludrocortisone (Florinef).

Notes About Fludrocortisone

- Fludrocortisone raises blood pressure by helping you to retain salt in your body and to discard potassium in your urine.
- Mild ankle swelling is common.
- Fludrocortisone usually is taken in the morning.
- Take fludrocortisone under close medical supervision.

Possible Side Effects

Swelling in the hands or feet, rapid weight gain, water retention, headache.

Diuretics

Patients who take prednisone may retain excess fluid in their bodies. Removing excess fluid also is helpful for lowering blood pressure. Diuretic medications (fluid pills) may be used briefly after transplantation to help you get rid of excess fluids caused by intravenous hydration during the surgery and while you were unable to eat. The most commonly used diuretics are furosemide (Lasix), hydrochlorothiazide (HCTZ), torsemide (Demadex), and bumetanide (Bumex). Spironolactone (Aldactone) may have been one of your diuretics before transplantation—this medication should be used very cautiously after transplantation.

Notes About Diuretics
- Take the diuretic early in the day so you will not have to get up several times a night to go to the bathroom.
- Taking a diuretic could cause your body to lose potassium. Potassium supplements may be prescribed for a short time to replenish the supply in your blood.
- Do not increase or decrease the dosage of your diuretic without consulting your transplant team.

Possible Side Effects
Low blood pressure, dizziness, lightheadedness, dehydration, more frequent urination, low potassium.

Cholesterol-Lowering Medications
Lowering your cholesterol may help prevent heart disease. People who have high cholesterol levels may be given medicine to lower it. The most commonly used cholesterol-lowering medicines are atorvastatin (Lipitor), simvastatin (Zocor), rosuvastatin (Crestor), pravastatin (Pravachol), and lovastatin (Mevacor). The primary immunosuppressive agents, cyclosporine and sirolimus, are the culprits causing high cholesterol and triglyceride levels in many patients who take them.

Notes About Cholesterol-Lowering Medications
- Cholesterol-lowering medicines usually are taken at night.
- The results of taking a cholesterol-lowering medication may not be seen for weeks or months.

- You will have blood tests while taking a cholesterol-lowering medicine to confirm that your liver is functioning normally and to monitor your cholesterol levels.
- Do not take a cholesterol-lowering medication if you are pregnant or considering pregnancy.
- Call the doctor who prescribed the cholesterol-lowering medication immediately if you experience muscle cramps or weakness, especially in your legs.

Possible Side Effects

Upset stomach, heartburn, change in the way foods taste, diarrhea, skin rash, headache, constipation, blurred vision, muscle damage.

Drug Interactions

Some medicines can interfere with the way cyclosporine, sirolimus, and tacrolimus are processed in your body and can lead to very high or very low blood levels of these drugs. This effect can result in toxicity or rejection of the transplanted liver. Be sure to discuss possible drug interactions with any physician who prescribes a new medicine for you. If you are unsure about a new medication, contact your transplant team.

Complications of Transplantation

Now that I am immunosuppressed, am I susceptible to infections?

What is chronic rejection?

Where can I learn more about organ transplantation?

More . . .

96. Now that I am immunosuppressed, am I susceptible to infections?

The antirejection medications that you are taking to prevent and treat rejection tell your immune system to accept your new organ. In doing so, they may also tell your immune system to accept other foreign invaders that it ordinarily would fight. As a consequence, taking antirejection medications can place you at greater risk for developing an infection. The most common infections result from viruses that have been lying dormant in your system or in the donated organ. To prevent infection, you will take antibacterial, antivirus, and antifungal medications for 3 to 6 months after your surgery.

If an infection is suspected, your caregivers may take sputum (the substance coughed up from your lungs), blood, and urine samples as well as samples from your catheter, wound, and drain sites. Signs that you may notice include fever, tiredness or fatigue, diarrhea or vomiting, redness or drainage around your incision or tube site, or a cough and sore throat. If an infection develops, it is treated with medication specific for the type of infection. The infectious disease specialist works with the transplant team to manage and treat infections. If an infection develops after you have been discharged from the hospital, it may be treated with antibiotics on an outpatient basis. However, some people need to be readmitted to the hospital for treatment with intravenous medications.

97. What is chronic rejection?

Chronic rejection (CR) involves progressive deterioration of the transplanted organ's function. The targets of the immune response are different from the targets in acute rejection. This damage occurs very slowly and

Chronic rejection

Occurs at least 3 months after transplant. It is a clinical and pathological diagnosis. There is progressive deterioration of the transplanted organ's function. Chronic rejection has features on tissue biopsy which are distinct from acute rejection, drug toxicity and other diseases.

is not a result of recurrent episodes of acute rejection. The main cause of CR, as with acute rejection, is too little immunosuppressive medication—either because the patient does not take his or her medications as prescribed or because the transplant physician reduces the dose in an attempt to avoid side effects. CR may be exacerbated by factors such as CMV infection, high cholesterol levels, diabetes, or hypertension.

Thanks to earlier recognition of acute and chronic rejection and the introduction of more powerful immunosuppressive agents (for example, tacrolimus and sirolimus), many of these cases can be successfully reversed.

98. Do I have to worry about long-term effects of immunosuppression?

The success of organ transplantation has resulted in longer survival after the operation for today's patients. This longer survival comes at a price, however: far more long-term complications than were seen in the past. More attention must therefore be paid to the long-term effects of the immunosuppressive drugs and their cumulative effects. For example, cyclosporine can cause hypertension and high cholesterol. Over the course of many years this combination results in heart attack and stroke. When expected survival after transplantation was short, these long-term issues were of minimal concern. Today, with longer survival being commonplace, heart disease is one of the major causes of death in transplant recipients.

The incidence of hypertension is attributed to the primary immunosuppressive agents. Standard antihypertensive medications are effective in treating this complication.

As noted earlier, over the long term hypertension can result in heart or vascular disease.

Obesity is another common problem after transplantation. Because many patients suffer from malnutrition before transplantation, these individuals are counseled to improve their nutrition afterward to help the healing process. Unfortunately, patients may become accustomed to this increased calorie intake and have a hard time cutting back their food consumption once recovery from surgery has been achieved. The subsequent obesity can decrease mobility and increase the risk of coronary artery disease.

Diabetes mellitus is frequently encountered in organ transplant recipients. Once again, the culprit is often the immunosuppressive agents, particularly tacrolimus and prednisone. The incidence of obesity correlates with diabetes incidence and both are cardiac risk factors.

Transplant-associated lymphoma is a feared complication of the immunosuppressive drugs. Fortunately, it occurs in only 1% to 2% of transplant recipients. This kind of lymphoma is associated with infection with the Epstein-Barr virus. Many patients who develop posttransplant lymphoproliferative disease (PTLD) can be treated with a reduction in immunosuppression, which may cause the PTLD to regress. In rare cases the PTLD becomes a true lymphoma and chemotherapy is required.

Transplant recipients have higher rates of both skin cancer and cervical cancer. Proper skin care, especially sun protection, is essential in these patients. For women, annual Pap smears are recommended.

99. I've heard that I might develop kidney problems after liver or heart transplantation. How can that happen?

Chronic renal failure is a recognized complication of all organ transplantation due to the need for immunosuppression. Both tacrolimus and cyclosporine can cause the kidneys to function less than optimally. Additionally, in patients with cirrhosis, heart disease, or renal disease before transplantation, the side effects of diuretic use, hypertension, and diabetes can all contribute to chronic renal failure in recipients of a new organ. Renal failure after the transplantation complicates medical management, leading to increased morbidity and mortality. The incidence of chronic renal disease among recipients of liver transplants is approximately 8% after 1 year, 14% after 3 years, and 18% after 5 years. For patients who have received a heart transplant, the incidence of chronic renal disease is 2% after 1 year, 7% after 3 years, and 11% after 5 years. This does not mean that all these patients need dialysis but rather that their kidneys are not fully functional. Some patients do, indeed, progress to dialysis; kidney transplantation may be indicated in these individuals.

A number of factors may predict the risk of developing renal failure, including age (older patients have a higher risk), gender (males have a higher risk than females), pretransplantation kidney function, and presence or absence of pretransplantation hypertension, diabetes, or hepatitis C infection. Overall, non-White, non-African American patients have the lowest risk of chronic renal failure.

Of course, most transplant recipients do *not* develop renal failure. For those with the risk factors mentioned previously, transplant physicians can work with them to reduce the risk of developing renal failure after organ transplantation. One technique is to reduce the dose of the primary immunosuppressive agent (that is, tacrolimus or cyclosporine). For those patients with a high risk or history of rejection, mycophenolate (Cell-Cept, Myfortic) can be added to the drug regimen. A recent addition to the immunosuppression armamentarium, sirolimus (Rapamycin, Rapamune), can also reduce the risk. Sirolimus is not toxic to the kidneys and may be used for primary immunosuppression. This drug cannot be used immediately after organ transplantation because it slows wound healing; instead, it is typically prescribed later if concerns about renal dysfunction arise.

100. Where can I learn more about organ transplantation?

Numerous resources are available to patients in need of organ transplantation and their families. You can obtain a wealth of information from your primary care physician, specialist, or local transplant center. Other resources are available through the Internet. Of course, be aware the quality of information on the websites varies widely. Here are some tips to help you evaluate a website:

- Check the "about us" section of the site. If there is no author listed or no credentials for the author, be suspicious.
- Check the attribution of the information. Experts have reviewed research in mainstream journals. Information from major government agencies, such as the U.S. Food and Drug Administration (FDA) and National Institutes of Health (NIH), has also been reviewed by experts. Information from drug companies may be reliable, but remember—these companies are in the business of selling products.

- Information put out by patient groups can be biased toward one point of view.
- Be wary of emotional testimonials. They can be misleading or irrelevant to you.
- Read many websites and cross-check what you find.
- If a treatment seems too good to be true, it probably is!
- Check with your primary care physician or transplant team before making any changes in your treatment plan based on information you found on the Internet.

Glossary

A

Antibiotics: medications prescribed to prevent and treat bacterial infections.

C

Cardiomyopathy: a weakening of the heart muscle due to inflammation ("myocarditis"), infections or viruses, alcohol abuse, the toxic effects of certain drugs, inherited or congenital heart problems, and "idiopathic" (unknown) causes.

Cardiorenal syndrome: also referred to as the heart–kidney syndrome. Syndrome in which any weakening in either condition adversely impacts the other's proper functioning, because the heart and kidneys need to maintain a delicate balance and have a carefully entwined relationship.

Chronic rejection: occurs at least 3 months after transplant. It is a clinical and pathological diagnosis. There is progressive deterioration of the transplanted organ's function. Chronic rejection has features on tissue biopsy which are distinct from acute rejection, drug toxicity and other diseases.

Cirrhosis: severe scarring of the liver. When normal liver tissue is damaged, it changes into scar tissue or fibrosis. This scar tissue can reduce blood flow through the liver, making it difficult for the liver to carry out functions that are essential for life and health. Many diseases and conditions may potentially cause severe scarring of the liver.

Coronary artery disease (CAD): the most common cause of heart failure caused by atherosclerosis (also called "hardening of the arteries"). This condition occurs when plaque (deposits of fat or cholesterol) accumulates on the inner surface of the arteries, narrowing the coronary arteries and reducing blood flow to the heart muscle. As a result, the heart muscle, deprived of oxygen-rich blood, cannot work normally and can weaken, and heart failure may develop.

Creatinine: blood test used as a marker of kidney function.

Crossmatch: a test that determines whether recipient cells and donor cells are compatible, carried out before transplant can take place.

D

Desensitization: a special medical treatment to try to remove donor-specific antibodies from the donor's blood whereby the recipient is treated with medication (intravenous immune globulin) to try to reduce the donor-specific antibodies.

Dialysis: a life-sustaining treatment that literally takes over the job of your kidneys. The two major types of dialysis are hemodialysis and peritoneal dialysis.

Directed donation: donated organs can be directed specifically to a transplant candidate on the rare occasion that a friend or family member of a transplant candidate may die during the waiting period. If the deceased becomes brain dead, his or her family may choose this option.

E

Ejection fraction (EF): a measure of how well the heart pumps blood out of its chambers (ventricles). With each contraction of your heart, a certain amount ("fraction") is pumped out of the heart ("ejected"). A normal ejection fraction is approximately 50% to 60%.

End-stage renal disease (ESRD): signals that the kidneys can no longer provide their vital functions, which include excreting toxins, managing electrolytes, and maintaining a proper fluid balance.

Endomyocardial biopsy: heart muscle biopsy after transplantation to monitor for rejection.

Engrafting: the process of induction therapy and maintenance therapy so your body accepts your kidney transplant.

F

Fulminant hepatic failure: a condition whereby a toxin (e.g., acetaminophen toxicity, mushroom poisoning) or virus (e.g., hepatitis A or hepatitis B) affects a previously healthy person with a normal liver. The risk of death from this condition is extremely high, and these patients take priority over the MELD scoring system to receive the next available liver from an acceptable blood type–matched donor.

G

Glomerular filtration rate (GFR): measure of the kidney's ability to filter. It gives us an estimate of what kind of a job your kidneys are doing.

H

Heart failure: a chronic condition in which your heart cannot supply enough blood and oxygen to your body to keep up with your body's demands. Sometimes called "congestive heart failure" because it is often associated with fluid buildup, swelling, and difficulty breathing.

Hemodialysis: a process in which a dialysis machine with a filter "cleans" your blood by removing toxins, correcting your electrolytes and removing excess fluid from your body.

Hemodynamics: pressures in each of your heart chambers and in your lungs (pulmonary artery pressure).

HLA, or human leukocyte antigen: these antigens are on leukocytes (white blood cells) and most solid tissues and organs of the body but are not present on red blood cells. They are the structures on the donor's transplanted organ that the recipients recognize as different from themselves and try to destroy. If donor and recipient have the same HLAs, there is less chance of rejection.

I

Immunosuppressive medications: also referred to as antirejection medications, these drugs are prescribed to help your immune system accept your new organ and are taken for the rest of your life.

Implanted cardioverter defibrillator (ICD): a small electronic device implanted permanently inside your body to continually monitor your heart rhythm (the pattern and speed of your heartbeat). If your heart rhythm becomes too slow or too fast, the ICD sends out electrical signals to restore your rhythm back to normal.

K

Kidneys: two bean-shaped organs located on either side of your spine that regulate the excretion of waste products and fluids, balance chemicals and minerals, and secrete hormones that affect the body's ability to

produce red blood cells and affect your blood pressure.

L

Live donor liver transplant (LDLT): the unique anatomy of the liver allows it to be separated into independent anatomic units that are able to retain their normal function. In these highly technical operations, the right lobe of the donor's liver (about 60% of the total liver) is implanted into the recipient. The recipient's entire liver is removed because it is diseased and functions poorly. After surgery, the rapid regeneration of the liver allows both the donor's and the recipient's livers to return to nearly full size.

Liver: the largest solid organ in the body, the liver performs more than 400 functions each day to keep the body healthy, such as use and storage of fats, sugars, iron, and vitamins; production of blood-clotting substances; detoxification of potentially harmful substances; and monitoring for the presence of bacteria in the blood.

M

MELD, Model for End-stage Liver Disease, score: a tool to rank patients on the liver transplant waiting list to assign cadaveric organs to those most in need of transplantation. The MELD score is actually a question that is answered by a mathematical calculation: "What is the risk of dying with liver disease in the next 3 months?"

Milan Criteria: developed in Milan, Italy, criteria to select patients with liver cancer to be viable candidates for transplantation. The Milan Criteria state that the patient with liver cancer has a low risk of recurrence after transplantation if there is a single tumor measuring less than or equal to 5 centimeters in diameter, or there are two or three tumors, each measuring less than 3 centimeters in diameter.

O

Organ procurement organization (OPO): private, nonprofit organizations in the United States that coordinate organ procurement in a designated service area, which may cover all or only part of a state. The OPO evaluates potential donors, discusses donation with potential donor family members, arranges for the surgical removal of donated organs, and arranges for the distribution of the organs according to national organ-sharing policies.

P

Paired exchange: a donor and recipient who are unable to donate because their blood types are incompatible or their immune systems were incompatible (they had a positive crossmatch) are evaluated and accepted into a participating transplant program to search for compatible matches.

Panel reactive antibody (PRA) test: a blood test performed before transplantation to determine if you have developed any antibodies to specific human antigens.

Peritoneal dialysis: a process by which your peritoneal membrane (the covering of your abdominal organs) acts as a filter. The abdominal cavity is filled with peritoneal dialysis fluid. The peritoneal membrane filters toxins and fluids from your blood into the peritoneal dialysis fluid. The peritoneal fluid containing the toxins is drained from your body after several hours and replaced with fresh peritoneal dialysis fluid. This procedure is called an exchange.

Portal hypertension: when pressure in the portal vein becomes elevated, due to a damaged liver.

Primary graft dysfunction: occurs when the transplanted heart fails for unknown reasons and isn't able to function, requiring urgent retransplantation to avoid patient death.

Primary graft nonfunction (PGNF): a condition that occurs within 1 week after organ transplantation. PGNF is not caused by rejection or blocked blood vessels; some transplanted organs do not work properly after surgery. These patients are usually in critical condition and experience organ failure within 48 hours after transplantation; they require immediate retransplantation and take priority over the MELD scoring system to receive the next available organ from an acceptable blood type–matched donor.

Pulmonary hypertension: high blood pressure in the arteries that supply the lungs.

R

Rejection: when your immune system attacks your transplant.

Renal failure: when the kidneys can no longer provide their vital functions.

T

Transplantation: surgical procedure in which a healthy organ from another person (donor) is placed into your body to assume the work of your nonfunctioning organ.

U

United Network for Organ Sharing (UNOS): a private, nonprofit organization that matches available organ donors with those awaiting transplantation. UNOS is under contract with the U.S. Department of Health and Human Services to maintain the nation's organ transplant waiting list. UNOS guarantees that all persons who need a transplant have an equal opportunity to receive their organs, regardless of age, gender, race, social status, and so on.

V

Vasoactive drugs: medications given to try to lower the pulmonary pressures or to increase the forward pumping force of the heart (the cardiac output). They are called vasoactive because they typically work by acting on the blood vessels in the body, typically dilating (enlarging) them, which can act to lower the pressure in the arteries.

Ventricular assist device (VAD): a mechanical pump device that is surgically implanted to help maintain the pumping ability of a heart that has become so severely weakened it is unable to effectively function on its own.

Glossary

Index

Index